Medicare HMOs

*Making Them
Work for the
Chronically Ill*

AHSR
HAP

Medicare HMOs

Making Them Work for the Chronically Ill

WITHDRAWN

Richard Kronick
Joy de Beyer

Gerard Anderson
Tony Dreyfus
Sontine Kalba
Mark McClellan
Mark Merlis
Thomas Rice

AHSR
HAP

Health Administration Press, Chicago, Illinois
Association for Health Services Research, Washington, DC

03   02   01   00   99   5   4   3   2   1

Library of Congress Cataloging-in-Publication Data

Kronick, Richard
   Medicare HMOs: making them work for the chronically ill / Richard Kronick and Joy de Beyer
      p.   cm.
   Includes bibliographical references and index.
   ISBN 1-56793-091-3 (alk. paper)
      1. Medicare. 2. Health maintenance organizations—United States. 3. Chronically ill—Medical care—United States—Finance. 4. Capitation fees (Medical care)—United States. 5. Adverse selection (Insurance)—United States. I. De Beyer, Joy. II. Title
RA412.3.K76   1998
362.1'04258—dc21   97-40045
                                                                         CIP

The paper used in this publication meets the minimum requirements of American National Standard for Information Sciences—Permanence of Paper for Printed Library Materials, ANSI Z39.48-1984.™

Health Administration Press
A division of the Foundation
   of the American College of
   Healthcare Executives
One North Franklin Street, Suite 1700
Chicago, IL 60606-3491
312/424-2800

Contents

List of Tables

List of Figures

Preface

In 1996, the Commonwealth Fund, as a complement to the extensive policy discussion and debate on risk-adjusted payment, provided a grant to Richard Kronick of the University of California at San Diego to explore the problems associated with risk selection and options that the Health Care Financing Administration may consider for addressing them. Under this grant, five papers were written and discussed at a seminar in Washington, D.C., on April 3, 1997. For this volume, the papers have been revised to take account of policy developments since the April 1997 conference, especially the passage of the Balanced Budget Act of 1997. This book also includes additional chapters on health-based payments, selection through disenrollment, and the feasibility of implementing proposed changes to provide a comprehensive discussion of strategies for addressing risk selection in Medicare. The final chapter synthesizes all of the proposed strategies and their feasibility, as well as the closing remarks by Bruce Vladeck, who was then completing his term as administrator of HCFA. The editors and authors are grateful to the Commonwealth Fund for the original project grant, Brian Biles for his encouragement, and Health Administration Press for their support in putting together this volume.

Richard Kronick
Joy de Beyer

Introduction and Overview

Richard Kronick and Joy de Beyer

A large and growing number of Medicare beneficiaries have joined health maintenance organizations (HMOs), paralleling trends in the under-65 population. At the beginning of 1998, 14 percent of all Medicare beneficiaries—more than 5.5 million people—received their Medicare benefits through a managed care plan (HCFA 1998), and in a number of populous California counties almost 50 percent of beneficiaries have joined an HMO. Further, the Balanced Budget Act (BBA), which was passed in August 1997, was intended to lead to additional increases in enrollment in managed care organizations. The BBA expanded the kinds of plans that can be offered to Medicare beneficiaries beyond traditional HMOs, dropped the restriction that no more than 50 percent of a plan's total enrollment be composed of Medicare beneficiaries, and made a number of other changes designed to increase the attractiveness of alternatives to fee-for-service Medicare.

It has been shown that HMOs can reduce the costs of providing healthcare to a defined population, increase quality of care, and lead to improved health outcomes. It is not at all clear, however, that HMOs that serve Medicare beneficiaries can be expected, in general, to achieve these desirable outcomes. HMOs are paid a fixed amount per month for each beneficiary, and although this payment is adjusted for age, gender, and other beneficiary characteristics, it is not adjusted for health status. As a result, HMOs are given strong financial incentives to avoid responsibility for the healthcare needs of those Medicare beneficiaries most in need of care. In addition, healthy beneficiaries are more attracted to HMOs than the less healthy, because the restrictions on access to care created by HMOs will be more worrisome for those expecting to use more healthcare services.

There is abundant evidence (summarized in Chapter 2) that HMOs have received a 'favorable selection' of Medicare beneficiaries—that is, those beneficiaries enrolled in HMOs have fewer expected healthcare needs than the beneficiaries remaining in fee-for-service plans. This favorable selection and the dynamics that lead to it create serious financial and quality of care concerns. The financial concerns arise because Medicare is paying more to the HMOs than it would be paying if beneficiaries remained in fee-for-service plans. The quality-of-care concerns arise because if HMOs are not rewarded for serving beneficiaries with greater-than-average expected healthcare needs, it is unlikely that the plans will develop systems of care that are responsive to those most in need.

This book describes and evaluates strategies designed to increase the likelihood that health plans serving Medicare beneficiaries will do a good job of providing healthcare to the beneficiaries most in need of care. This introductory chapter describes the large and growing role of HMOs in the Medicare program, defines risk selection and explains the problems associated with it, and outlines the material covered in subsequent chapters.

HMOs AND THE MEDICARE PROGRAM

It is only fairly recently that HMOs have begun to play a significant role in managing and delivering care for Medicare beneficiaries. Although the first managed care demonstrations began in 1982, enrollment grew slowly at first. The growth rate has rapidly increased over the past five years, however. Figure 1.1 shows Medicare managed care enrollment growth. Since 1992, Medicare enrollment in risk-contract HMOs has more than tripled (HCFA 1997). The Congressional Budget Office projects that enrollment in risk-contract HMOs will exceed one-third of all beneficiaries within 10 years (cited in Lamphere et al. 1997). In February 1998, there were 338 plans with Medicare risk contracts. Figure 1.2 shows the number of plans in December each year from 1985 through 1997. Managed care expenditures accounted for $19.1 billion (9.3 percent) of the total $206 billion in Medicare benefit payments in fiscal year 1996 (Dallek and Swirsky 1997).

Managed care plans are able to participate in the Medicare program through three types of contracts—risk, cost, and healthcare prepayment plans (HCPPs)—and through various demonstration projects. Risk plans are paid using the AAPCC, a per-capita premium set at approximately 95 percent of

Figure 1.1 Medicare Risk Contract/Managed Care Enrollment (1985 to 1997)

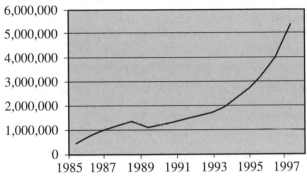

Note: These figures include all risk contracts, including demonstrations. They exclude cost contracts and HCPPs. Figures are for December of each year.

Source: HCFA, Medicare Contract and State Summary Reports—Monthly. Feb 1998.

Figure 1.2 Managed Care Plans Participating in the Medicare Risk Contract Programs (1985 to 1997)

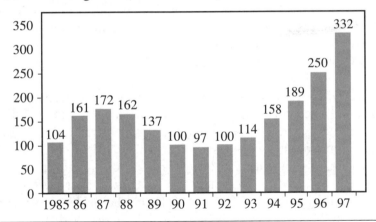

Note: These figures include all risk contracts, including demonstrations. They exclude cost contracts and HCPPs. Figures are for December of each year.

Source: HCFA, Medicare Contract and State Summary Reports—Monthly. Feb 1998.

the projected average expenses for fee-for-service beneficiaries in a given county, which takes into account age, gender, welfare status, and institutional status. Medicare HMO capitation rates approximate what a group of HMO enrollees would have cost under fee-for-service, with a small downward adjustment to account for the savings expected from managed care. Risk plans must provide all Medicare-covered services and assume full financial risk for these services. Most plans offer additional services such as prescription drugs and eyeglasses. Cost contracts now cover less than 2 percent of all Medicare beneficiaries and are being phased out. Risk contracts dominate Medicare managed care and are the focus of this book.

If biased selection exists and the medical care needs of HMO enrollees differ from average Medicare beneficiaries of similar age, gender, and other characteristics accounted for in the AAPCC, then the premiums paid to HMOs will not, on average, reflect the costs of caring for their enrollees. If HMO enrollees have greater needs for care than average, then the HMO has an adverse selection of risk and will lose money under the AAPCC payment formula. If HMO enrollees have less need for medical care than the average in the group on which capitation is based, then the HMO has a favorable selection of risk, and the AAPCC pays more than would have been spent by Medicare if the HMO beneficiaries had remained in fee-for-service. Further, if HMOs receive a favorable selection, then the beneficiaries remaining in fee-for-service will be more expensive than average, and the AAPCC will increase in subsequent years, thus increasing the extent of overpayments. Overpayments to HMOs waste taxpayers' money and lead to increased financial pressure on the Medicare Trust Fund and on the general revenues used to pay for Part B services. The reasons for encouraging the growth of Medicare HMOs are savings and the potential to improve quality, not to pay more money to health plan administrators and providers than would have been paid under fee-for-service. Thus, biased selection raises a serious financial issue.

Of greater concern to many, however, is the effect of the dynamics that lead to biased selection on the quality of care for those Medicare beneficiaries who are most in need of care—the chronically ill, the severely disabled, and those with a variety of serious medical problems. Part of the promise of managed care is that it will create healthcare delivery systems that are more responsive to the needs of consumers than was true under fee-for-service. However, in the current environment, an HMO that seeks to excel in providing care to beneficiaries with cancer, heart disease or diabetes, or that seeks aggressively to recruit the most respected subspecialists in the community, would likely cause its own demise. It would attract an unfavorable selection of risk, be paid less than it needs to provide care to its enrollees, and be forced either to change course or go out of business.[1]

The financial imperative for HMOs to avoid attracting an adverse selection of enrollees makes one fear that HMOs will not develop systems of care responsive to those individuals who are most in need of care, and that these individuals will be poorly served in HMOs and will face increasingly steep Medigap premiums (or high out-of-pocket payments) if they choose to stay in fee-for-service. The purpose of insurance is to spread risk among the healthy and the sick; the dynamic of risk selection defeats that purpose and threatens the quality of care available to those most in need.

Many analysts assert, and we agree, that changing the HMO payment system to adjust payments based on the health status of enrollees is the most effective action that the Health Care Financing Administration (HCFA) could take to limit the financial pressures and quality-of-care concerns created by risk-selection dynamics. Beginning in 2000, as required under the Balanced Budget Act, HCFA will begin using inpatient data to make health-based payment adjustments to HMOs. Health-based payment (also known as risk-adjusted payment) would remove some of the incentive to plans to avoid high-risk beneficiaries by paying plans a premium commensurate with the costs of caring for high-risk enrollees. In addition, because health-based payment systems pay plans a reduced premium for healthier enrollees who are at lower risk for needing costly care, these low-risk enrollees become much less profitable to the plan. Payments based on enrollee health or risk status remove some of the financial imperative of plans to attract a biased set of enrollees.

Health-based payment is necessary, but it is not sufficient to create an environment that will limit risk selection and encourage the development of delivery systems that provide high-quality care to those Medicare beneficiaries most in need. Available health-based payment systems would differentiate among groups of enrollees with particular health problems or health status but would pay the same for everyone within a particular health-status group. No group would be homogeneous, so insurers would still have an incentive to selectively enroll some members and avoid others within any risk group. Imagine a group of beneficiaries, each of whom has congestive heart failure and diabetes. If an HMO received an identical payment for each enrolled member of the group, the plan would still be able to profit if it could attract those beneficiaries who need less care than the average member of the group. Because health-based payments are not sufficient to solve completely the problems associated with risk selection, this book proposes complementary strategies that would help decrease the extent to which beneficiaries with high risk will want to stay away from HMOs and make it harder for plans to avoid the high-risk members of a particular risk group.

CHAPTER SUMMARIES

Chapter 2 reviews the evidence about the extent of risk selection in the Medicare program and describes why and how risk selection occurs. Factors that limit the ability of HMOs to attempt to select favorable risks are considered, and the extent to which risk selection is likely to remain a problem in mature Medicare HMO markets is discussed.

Chapter 3 asserts that adjusting HMO capitation payments to reflect health status is the most effective strategy to reduce the extent of risk selection and improve quality of care for the chronically ill. Anthony Dreyfus and Richard Kronick describe the rationale for health-based payments, HCFA's strategy for implementing health-based payment, and the obstacles to successful implementation. They suggest a variety of strategies for overcoming these obstacles.

Chapter 4 explains why it is so important for Medicare beneficiaries to be provided with timely, comprehensive, objective, comparative information on their choices under Medicare. The BBA mandates that information be given and provides some funding to do so, but the act will also increase the complexity of choices by introducing new options. The options for Medicare coverage are described, as well as the kinds of information now available to beneficiaries and the regulation of that information. Mark Merlis discusses the key issues that must be considered in delivering information to Medicare beneficiaries, including what beneficiaries want and need to know to make informed choices among plans, and methods of communicating that information to beneficiaries. Finally, the chapter assesses the likely effect of better beneficiary information, especially its potential effect on risk selection.

Chapter 5 describes the current enrollment system for HMOs and Medigap supplementary policies and the problems associated with that process. The BBA requires that there be coordinated, annual open enrollment for HMOs; Tom Rice discusses the relative merits and disadvantages of equalizing the rules for HMOs and Medigap policies and of using independent brokers to handle enrollment.

Wide variation in health plan offerings is one of the reasons for the complexity of choice among HMOs and fee-for-service Medicare. In Chapter 6, Mark McClellan and Sontine Kalba weigh the tradeoffs between standardized benefit packages and diversity among health plan offerings. In light of recent private sector experiences with standardizing benefit packages, the authors assess the current extent of HMO benefit package diversity in Medicare and discuss key issues for reforming Medicare plan choice and plan diversity and the likely consequences for risk selection and Medicare costs.

Chapter 7 makes a case for stronger oversight and additional regulation of HMO plans participating in Medicare. Gerard Anderson describes the use of services by Medicare beneficiaries with chronic illnesses, as well as the legislative and regulatory actions that some states have taken to improve the care that HMOs provide to people with special healthcare needs. He recommends ways for Medicare to strengthen oversight of marketing and some additional service and care requirements that could make Medicare plans more responsive to high-need beneficiaries.

Evidence exists that disenrollment from Medicare HMOs is selective of beneficiaries with relatively high healthcare needs, and it worsens risk selection. Because the actions—or inaction—of HMOs may in part be responsible for this, disenrollment is an area for policy review. Chapter 8 summarizes studies of the extent and causes of disenrollment, describes the present system for monitoring and publicizing disenrollment data, and discusses how the restrictions that the BBA gradually introduces on disenrollment may affect the picture.

Chapter 9 reviews some of the key relevant reforms of the Medicare program that are already on HCFA's agenda, including those mandated under the Balanced Budget Act of 1997, and summarizes the additional strategies for addressing risk selection that are suggested in this book. Factors affecting the political, economic, and technical feasibility of implementing the proposed strategies are explored: cost, whether the actions needed from HCFA would be deemed acceptable and appropriate, whether vested interests would be threatened, and whether the knowledge and techniques exist to implement the strategies effectively. Finally, in recognition of the resource and other constraints within which HCFA operates, we single out the actions that we think should have the highest priority, applying the criteria of feasibility and likelihood of making the biggest improvement in the problems associated with risk selection.

NOTE

1. See Jones 1996 for a clear statement of this problem.

REFERENCES

Dallek, G., and L. Swirsky. 1997. *Comparing Medicare HMOs: Do They Keep Their Members?* Washington, DC: Families USA Foundation.

Health Care Financing Administration (HCFA). 1997. "Managed Care in Medicare and Medicaid." Fact Sheet. http://www.hcfa.gov/facts/f960900.htm. Feb. 1998.

Health Care Financing Administration (HCFA). 1998. "Medicare Managed Care Monthly Reports." http://www.hcfa.gov/stats/monthly.htm. Feb. 1998.

Jones, S. 1996. "Why Not the Best for the Chronically Ill?" *Health Insurance Reform Project Research Agenda Brief.* George Washington University.

Lamphere, J. A., P. Newhouse, K. Langwell, and D. Sherman. 1997. "The Surge in Medicare Managed Care: An Update." *Health Affairs* 16 (3): 127–33.

The Problem of Selection in Medicare Risk-Contract HMOs

Richard Kronick and Joy de Beyer

C oncern about risk selection began with the first evaluation of the risk program in the 1980s and persists even in mature markets where HMO penetration rates have reached 40 or 50 percent. This chapter reviews published estimates of the magnitude of risk selection and analyzes the mechanisms and processes through which selection occurs as a prelude to the discussion in the rest of the book on ways to address selection.

HOW BIG A PROBLEM IS RISK SELECTION IN MEDICARE HMOs?

The size of the cost and quality problem posed by risk selection partly depends on the extent of selection bias. At least 20 studies have measured selection bias in Medicare HMOs, using three sets of indicators: health status, mortality rates, and pre-enrollment service utilization or cost.[1] Some studies compare pre-enrollment utilization and expenditure data for HMO enrollees and beneficiaries in fee-for-service, while others gather information through surveys of enrollees and a control group of fee-for-service beneficiaries. Typically, when comparing HMO enrollees with groups in fee-for-service Medicare, studies control for the demographic adjustors included in the AAPCC, because these are taken into account in setting HMO payment rates. The overwhelming predominance of evidence is that there is substantial favorable selection for which the AAPCC does not adjust.

Controlling for demographic characteristics, Medicare HMO enrollees are found to be, on average, healthier than beneficiaries in fee-for-service. They have a lower prevalence of chronic conditions, better self-reported health status, and better functional health status (Lichtenstein et al. 1991; Lichtenstein et al. 1992; Brown et al. 1993; Garfinkel et al. 1986; Riley et al. 1996; Rodgers and Smith 1996; Dowd et al. 1996). HMOs appear to have done particularly well in avoiding very disabled enrollees.

Five studies comparing age-adjusted mortality rates between HMOs and fee-for-service Medicare report at least 20 to 30 percent less mortality among HMO enrollees than among Medicare fee-for-service beneficiaries (USGAO 1986; PPRC 1996; Brown et al. 1993; Riley, Lubitz, and Rabey 1991).[2] As a result of the concentration of Medicare expenditures in the last year of life, even small differences in mortality rates of beneficiaries in HMOs compared to beneficiaries in fee-for-service have large effects on expected resource needs: if the age-adjusted mortality rate in HMOs is 25 percent lower than in fee-for-service, we would expect total HMO expenditures, other things being equal, to be approximately 5.7 percent below the fee-for-service level.[3]

Pre-enrollment costs and use of services are consistently found to be lower for HMO enrollees than for Medicare recipients who remain in fee-for-service (Eggers and Prihoda 1982; Porell and Turner 1990; Lichtenstein et al. 1992; Brown et al. 1993; Dowd et al. 1994; PPRC 1996). Brown et al.'s (1993) comparison of prior-year Medicare claims data for 1990 of 6,476 risk HMO enrollees and 6,381 fee-for-service beneficiaries remains the most comprehensive and influential study of selection. They found that in the year prior to enrolling, HMO enrollees' health costs were 23 percent lower than for fee-for-service beneficiaries. Expected costs during the first year of enrollment were 10.7 percent below a demographically similar fee-for-service group. Thus, they estimated that Medicare capitation payments at 95 percent of the fee-for-service average cost were 5.7 percent higher than the hypothetical fee-for-service cost would have been. A more recent analysis of fee-for-service spending during the six months prior to enrollment for a 5 percent sample of HMO enrollees between 1989 and 1994 found even larger effects: pre-enrollment spending for HMO enrollees was 37 percent lower than spending for beneficiaries who remained in fee-for-service (PPRC 1996).

Contrary data and opinions exist on whether HMOs have favorable selection. A little evidence has been found that some HMOs have experienced adverse selection: for example, Brown et al. (1993) found adverse enrollment in 1 of 17 plans studied, and inconclusive evidence for two others. Analysis commissioned by the HMO industry questions whether favorable selection persists as HMO enrollees age and the risk-contract market grows and matures.[4] Using the 1992 (round 4) Medicare Current Beneficiary Survey (MCBS), Rodgers and Smith (1996) found higher proportions of younger and healthy people and also of chronically ill and lower income Medicare beneficiaries in HMOs than in a carefully matched fee-for-service group; they estimated that these mixed selection effects cancelled out to make overall average cost of care about the same in fee-for-service as in HMOs (after controlling for demographic factors in the AAPCC). However, these conclusions are undermined by small sample size and other sampling and methodological problems.[5] Moreover, more recent comparable data from the 1994 (round 10) MCBS showed that HMO enrollee costs were only 85 percent of the predicted costs of fee-for-service beneficiaries (Riley et al. 1996). The HMO sample had better self-reported and functional health status and lower prevalence of chronic conditions.

Most studies report on selection in markets with relatively low levels of Medicare HMO penetration, because until recently almost all markets had relatively low Medicare HMO enrollment. However, just as strong favorable selection seems to exist among new enrollees in markets with relatively high Medicare penetration (25 percent or more of beneficiaries in HMOs) as in markets with low HMO penetration (Nelson et al. 1996). And even in the more mature California market, where close to 50 percent of the Medicare beneficiaries in some counties are enrolled in HMOs, substantial risk selection continues to exist among new enrollees (USGAO 1997).

Of greater concern than the financial implications of risk selection, the financial imperatives to obtain a favorable selection of risks (relative to the capitation) threaten the quality of care for HMO enrollees with the greatest healthcare needs. Less has been published on this topic, and the evidence comparing healthcare quality and outcomes between fee-for-service and HMOs is mixed. A variety of studies find that beneficiary satisfaction is similar in HMOs and fee-for-service, and that quality of care and outcomes for average beneficiaries is also similar.[6] However, results appear to be less positive for some high-need beneficiaries. Ware et al. (1996) found that health outcomes of elderly patients worsened under managed care compared to fee-for-service; Shaugnessey, Schlenker, and Hittle (1994) found that HMOs provide much less home health care than recipients receive in fee-for-service, and that health outcomes suffer as a result. A third study found that stroke patients treated in Medicare HMOs were less likely to be discharged to rehabilitation facilities and more likely to be discharged to nursing homes than were similar patients in fee-for-service (Retchin et al. 1997). Other research has found that rehabilitation services have a better success rate than nursing homes in restoring functional abilities of stroke patients and enabling them to return to the community (cited in Komisar, Hunt-McCool, and Feder 1997/98). On the other hand, long-term survival in two Medicare HMOs was at least as good as, and possibly better than, outcomes in the fee-for-service system for a sample of 13,358 women over age 65 diagnosed with breast cancer between 1985 and 1992, and the use of recommended therapy for early-stage breast cancer was more frequent in the two HMOs (Potosky et al. 1997). Much more work is needed here, but there is enough evidence to justify the theoretical concern: HMOs, in the current environment, are not rewarded for excellence in providing care to the chronically ill. It appears that many HMOs have responded to these incentives as we would expect and have not worked hard to develop systems of care that are responsive to those most in need.

In summary, the overwhelming evidence is that HMOs, on average, enjoy favorable selection that has resulted in Medicare paying them more than the enrollees would have cost had they remained in fee-for-service. Enrollment data show that the most vulnerable subgroups—the old elderly, the disabled, and the chronically ill—are less likely to join HMOs than other Medicare beneficiaries. It is unclear whether the most needy are poorly served in Medicare HMOs, but there is some evidence to suggest that they are. In order to assure that rapidly growing Medicare HMO enrollment promotes the development of high-quality care for those most in need, risk selection and the dynamics that create it are policy problems requiring solutions.

HOW AND WHY RISK SELECTION OCCURS

Understanding how and why risk selection can occur is important for evaluating which policies may be effective in solving the problem. It is well known that among almost any group of people, approximately 20 percent of the group can be expected to account for 80 percent of group expenditures. Some people need a lot of care; most need little or none. This characteristic gives plans a strong incentive to attract the healthy majority and avoid the sickest people. Selection bias can arise from deliberate or inadvertent actions by health plans, as well as from patterns of consumer choice. It can occur either at the time of enrollment or through disenrollment of plan members who are above the group average; each of these possibilities require different policy responses.

Selection at Enrollment

Beneficiary preferences

In deciding whether to enroll in an HMO, beneficiaries weigh costs, the benefit package, and access to particular providers and facilities. They balance the potential for saving money, reducing paperwork, and having all care coordinated through one set of providers against the loss of freedom of choosing their provider and concerns about not being able to obtain needed care (or increased hassles associated with obtaining this care). Consumer choice will cause risk selection if HMOs intrinsically appeal more to healthier people.

The main incentive for beneficiaries to join an HMO is to save money[7]— in some areas of the country, HMOs offer a package of supplemental benefits for zero premium that may cost $1,500 or more per year if purchased as a Medigap policy. The relationship between health status and financial benefit from joining an HMO is quite different for those with and without supplementary insurance. Among beneficiaries with Medigap policies currently in fee-for-service who are deciding whether to switch to an HMO with similar coverage, the financial benefit from joining an HMO is similar for those who are sicker and those who are healthier. However, for people who are without supplemental coverage choosing between an HMO and fee-for-service Medicare, the potential savings from joining a zero premium HMO increase as health status deteriorates because of the potentially large copayments, deductibles, and uncovered services in fee-for-service.

The main disincentives to enrolling in an HMO are loss of freedom to choose a provider, obstacles that may be placed in the way of obtaining medically necessary care, and, potentially, denial of coverage for care in the HMO that may have been paid for in fee-for-service. These considerations are much more important to those with high healthcare needs or risks. Sicker people tend to have strong established relationships with healthcare providers (especially their physicians), which they are reluctant to give up. A required switch to unfamiliar new providers is a strong deterrent to enrolling in an HMO (Berki and Ashcroft 1980; Billi et al. 1993). The greater a person's healthcare needs, the greater the number of physicians who may be providing care and the less likely it is that all physicians will be in a single HMO. Even if a particular HMO does include all of the physicians, beneficiaries may worry that the HMO utilization review process will impede obtaining needed care, and the weight of these concerns is likely to increase as the expected need for care increases.

For beneficiaries who have a Medigap policy, the drawbacks of managed care are higher for those with heavier needs while the monetary benefits of joining do not differ for the healthy and the sick, so it makes sense to expect that those with heavier needs are less likely to join an HMO than beneficiaries with fewer healthcare needs. For the 11 percent of beneficiaries who lack supplemental coverage, both the costs and benefits of joining an HMO are expected to be greater for beneficiaries with heavy needs than for beneficiaries with lighter needs; the net expected effect on the direction and extent of selection bias for these beneficiaries is ambiguous.[8, 9]

Because most beneficiaries do have supplemental coverage, we would expect favorable selection to HMOs from beneficiary enrollment decisions even if HMOs were trying as hard as possible to provide excellent care to those most in need. However, we have created a system in which it is not reasonable to expect plans to strive for excellence in the care of the chronically ill, and so the expected selection effects from consumer preferences will only be aggravated by HMO actions.

Actions by plans

Attempting to attract a healthy, lower-risk group and to avoid an adverse selection of risk is sound business practice in a competitive managed care market in which payments are not adjusted for enrollee health status. HMOs could use a variety of strategies to influence enrollment decisions:

- marketing to the healthy;
- benefit packages tailored to attract low-risk people;
- provider networks designed to minimize involvement of the specialists who treat costly conditions;
- limiting service availability in very low income areas;
- prior approval requirements that increase the "hassle factor" the most for those who use the most healthcare; and
- utilization review processes that target those services, such as home health care and durable medical equipment, that are heavily used by the chronically ill.

Although HCFA tries to prevent skimming by plans through its review process when an HMO applies for a risk contract and through subsequent review and approval of marketing materials, HMOs still have many opportunities to influence the composition of their enrollment. There are many anecdotes about plan strategic behavior, mostly focused on marketing practices, but little systematic study exists. Thus, although there is much opportunity for plans to take actions to influence selection, we emphasize that there is relatively little evidence about the extent to which plans systematically engage in these actions.

Marketing

Both generic marketing strategies and specific enrollment techniques can be used to influence selection. The generic strategies aim marketing materials at the healthy, while the specific seek out healthy people and try to avoid the sick or disabled. Marketing opportunities to appeal to selected target groups remain despite HCFA reviews of all HMO marketing and rules intended to ensure that no groups of Medicare beneficiaries are systematically excluded or differentially courted. Pictures of active, healthy seniors in media advertisements may give the message to those who are sick that the HMO is not for them. Many TV and print ads for Medicare senior products show beneficiaries playing golf or strolling hand-in-hand on a tranquil river bank. Few depict people with quadriplegia, or heart attack or stroke victims. Advertisements rarely trumpet an HMO as the best place to be if you are really sick. However, a study in 1987–1989 of the marketing activities of 22 HMOs (including review of materials and interviews with HMO staff) concluded that it was unlikely that there was any systematic marketing or market segmentation responsible for the favorable risk selection that was found (Lichtenstein et al. 1992).

Few marketing materials are targeted at the under-65 Medicare disabled, and many Medicare products have names that suggest that the under-65 are not welcome: Health 65, 65 Plus, Secure Horizons, Senior Advantage, Senior Care, Senior Choice, Senior Plan, Senior Plus. It is not surprising that the under-65 disabled are seriously underrepresented in HMOs,[10] given this marketing bias and all the other reasons that may make HMOs unattractive to this group.

In addition to generic methods of attracting the fit and discouraging the sick, plans can actively discourage enrollment of sick beneficiaries. Although prohibited by Medicare from health screening, there are reports of HMOs that provide potential enrollees with physical examinations one month before enrollment (billed to Medicare under fee-for-service), which is strongly suggestive of screening (USGAO 1986). A 1993 Health and Human Services survey of nearly 3,000 Medicare beneficiaries found "serious problems with enrollment procedures and service access . . .": 43 percent of individuals were asked about their health status when applying to a HMO, and 3 percent were required to have a physical before joining. The report did not cite direct contravention of the regulation but noted that the survey suggests "the possibility of health screening and selective enrollment" (Kertesz 1995). For many of the sick and chronically ill, subtle health screening tools are not needed; a face-to-face meeting with a marketer would be enough to identify elevated levels of need. While marketers should present both the pros and cons of joining, a slight shading of the pros and cons when presenting to a person who is sick may be enough to create substantial selection effects.

HCFA discourages but does not prohibit marketing by providers, and, in any case, providers are likely to be asked their advice and opinions about alternative healthcare options. Physicians are in a very powerful position to influence choice and have extensive information on their patients' health status. If providers participate in several plans or both fee-for-service Medicare and HMOs, maximizing their own compensation would likely mean steering high users to fee-for-service and healthier patients to HMOs. And even if they act entirely in their patients' best interests, they may advise patients with multi-system problems to avoid plans that have limited choice of specialists or may believe that higher risk patients will be better cared for under fee-for-service. Concern about selection initiated by providers will grow as providers are increasingly put at risk. This is already a trend in California, where it is becoming common for HMOs to pass risk on to provider groups. The new "Medicare+Choice" options introduced by the BBA enables provider groups to contract directly with HCFA to care for Medicare beneficiaries on a capitated basis. Physicians who have a stake in these provider-sponsored networks (PSNs) will have the same incentives as HMOs to avoid high-risk beneficiaries, and their detailed information on the health status and medical histories of their own patients will put them in a highly privileged position, which they could use to steer their sicker patients into traditional Medicare and those who are healthier into their PSOs.

Benefits

Plans can tailor benefits to attract the healthy or to deter the sick. For example, they can provide a broad array of preventive care but relatively little coverage of prescription drugs or long-term care. The medical director of one large health plan wrote that changes in their benefit packages had "been designed to attract and keep healthy people within the pool of the insured" (Maurer 1990). Discouraging unhealthy enrollees is a corollary of attracting healthy ones. One HMO trade publication carried an article explicitly recommending that health plans identify characteristics in groups that produce losses and reposition their products to discourage those people from enrolling (Edres and Gunter, cited in Newhouse 1994).

However, coverage limitations in the basic Medicare benefit package and fierce competition among Medicare HMOs in many markets have led to HMO benefit offerings that, relative to fee-for-service, should be attractive to those in greater need. Many HMOs offer supplemental benefits, particularly prescription drug coverage, that are attractive to high users. Further, in the markets with the highest Medicare HMO enrollment, competitive pressures have created an environment in which most plans offer similar supplemental benefits packages. In these markets, HMOs frequently tinker with benefit packages as they jockey with each other for market share; for example, if one HMO improves its dental benefits, others in the area are likely to follow suit quickly. Little direct evidence exists of similar behavior of tailoring packages to make them less attractive to the chronically ill.

Indirect evidence of benefit package tailoring can be seen from consideration of the types of policies that are *not* offered. For example, most beneficiaries in HMOs have prescription drug coverage, and this coverage typically pays for prescriptions (after a relatively small deductible) up to a maximum of some amount (e.g., $1,500 per year). One does not find HMOs offering actuarially equivalent policies with a very high deductible for prescription drugs (e.g., $2,000 per year) but that pay for most of the costs beyond the deductible level. Given a hypothesis of risk-aversion among beneficiaries, a high-deductible catastrophic policy should be more attractive than an actuarially equivalent policy that leaves beneficiaries with unlimited exposure to catastrophic expenses. The absence of catastrophic policies may reflect HMO judgment about beneficiary myopia, but more likely it reflects concerns about unfavorable risk selection. Similarly, many beneficiaries may prefer coverage of additional home health care services to an actuarially equivalent policy that covers preventive services; however, concerns about adverse selection are very likely part of the reason that such policies are not available.

An additional concern about the diversity of benefit packages exists: namely, that a plethora of choices is confusing to beneficiaries. It is difficult for beneficiaries to gather and assess information about their HMO choices in many markets. Efforts to compile side-by-side comparison charts of HMOs are underway, but even where these exist they are not widely distributed, and most beneficiaries do not know about them. So a beneficiary who is thinking about joining an HMO would have to know that they could call a toll-free number or an information, counseling, and assistance (ICA) program to get a list of available HMOs in their area. Then they would have to call each HMO to request information. One of the authors attempted this for San Diego and Los Angeles. It took two hours of phone calls, and then only about half of the information packages that were promised actually arrived. It is difficult to compare plans because formats, terminology, and level of detail are not standardized.[11]

Older adults find it more difficult than young people to process and assimilate unfamiliar, difficult material, and many Medicare beneficiaries are hampered by physical or mental frailty or poor vision or hearing.[12] Some beneficiaries will need written materials to be in a large typeface, or pitched at a sixth-grade reading level. The information problem is proportional to the number of plans on offer, differing in benefits, exclusions, and rules. The frailest and sickest people may have the most difficulty in gathering, comparing, and processing information. And because it is those who have the greatest need who are likely to be most reluctant to leave fee-for-service to begin with, high information cost is likely to have more effect on the decisions of the sick than on the decisions of the healthy. The BBA requires HCFA to provide comparative information on their Medicare choices to each beneficiary each year; depending on the quality, completeness, and simplicity of the information, this problem will be attenuated (see Chapter 4 for details).

Access to care: provider networks and facilities and utilization review practices

The composition of a plan's provider network and the places where that care is provided can have a powerful effect on who enrolls. Plans can avoid the providers who specialize in treating costly conditions.[13] They can avoid providers who practice in low-income areas, where the burden of illness is likely to be high. They can recruit newly trained specialists with limited patient following rather than more experienced specialists who may bring with them large numbers of patients in need of specialized (expensive) care. Evidence of plans tailoring their networks to avoid high-risk members is limited. Academic health centers, inner-city physicians, and the occasional highly visible specialist complain about difficulty in joining HMO networks, but it is not clear whether there is a systematic problem that needs an aggressive solution.

The barriers that HMOs set up to limit care do appear to disproportionately affect the choices made by the chronically ill and those people most in need of health services. If, for example, a primary care physician referral to a specialist needs to be re-authorized after every three visits to the specialist, then an extra hurdle is created for the chronically ill. There is strong evidence that HMOs provide much less home health care than recipients receive in fee-for-service and that health outcomes suffer as a result (Shaugnessey, Schlenker, and Hittle 1994; Nelson et al. 1996). Although a similar study of durable medical equipment (DME) has not been performed, sharp reductions in access to DME in HMOs are likely as well. Conversely, there are relatively few examples of HMOs making large investments in developing systems of care that are especially responsive to individuals most in need of health services. Determining what to do about these problems is difficult—we turn to HMOs in an attempt to get better value for money, and this means that we expect that some services that are provided in fee-for-service will not be provided in HMOs. The services that are eliminated, however, should be services that do not improve beneficiary quality of life; some evidence exists that the elimination of some HMO services results in poorer outcomes, particularly for people most in need. We return to this problem when considering credentialing of health plans below.

Risk Selection at Disenrollment

Risk selection can occur not only because those beneficiaries who enroll in HMOs are different from beneficiaries who do not enroll, but also because those who disenroll are different from those who remain. Chapter 8 summarizes the existing data on the magnitude of and trends in disenrollment and reviews the evidence for the extent to which selective disenrollment further exacerbates risk selection in Medicare HMOs. Disenrollees have been found to be of significantly higher risk than those who remain, measuring disability and health status, functional impairment, service utilization, risk factors, and mortality (Rossiter et al. 1989; Tucker and Langwell 1988; Langwell and Hadley 1989; Riley, Rabey, and Kasper 1989; Adams and Tyler 1995).

Consumer preferences

Consumer preferences, unmediated by plan actions, are likely to have a mixed selection effect on disenrollment. Health plan enrollees who are sicker have more opportunities to test and be dissatisfied with the HMO, and thus may be more likely to disenroll. Similarly, enrollees with greater needs for care may be more likely to want care from a provider who is not in the HMO, and thus may be more likely to disenroll. However, the sick will also be using more healthcare and should be forming stronger attachments to providers, as well as benefiting more from coordination and reduced paperwork, which should make beneficiaries more likely to stay enrolled when sick. Certainly the sick should be less likely than the healthy to switch to another HMO for a lower premium. But if the plan does not perform well, high-use beneficiaries will become dissatisfied more quickly and will be more likely to return to fee-for-service. A clear difference exists between the consumer preference selection effects at enrollment and disenrollment: disenrollment is likely to be selective of the sick only if the HMO performs poorly, but sick people are less likely to enroll in an HMO almost regardless of how welcoming the plan is to them because those who are already sick are more likely to have to change provider relationships or to fear intrusive utilization review.

Plan actions

If plan enrollees who are heavy service users receive systematically less attention or poorer care than light users, or if they must contend with onerous grievance processes, substantial selective disenrollment may occur, as those most in need of care disproportionately leave. Selective disenrollment is a potentially powerful device for selection, because enrollees' health status is generally known to the plan and high-risk individuals can be targeted directly. There is no documented evidence of HMOs deliberately encouraging high-risk people to disenroll, but a number of standard HMO practices can be expected to affect high users selectively. A 1993 study of disenrollees from HMOs in Los Angeles found numerous examples of egregious practice—denial or very long delays in care or services, until beneficiaries opted out of the HMO, sometimes as a last resort (Dallek et al. 1993).

Limits on HMO Incentives to Select Favorable Risks

We have discussed a variety of actions that HMOs may take to influence the composition of their enrollment. But there are forces that restrain plans from acting aggressively to improve their mix of risks:

- The marketing department wants to enroll as many beneficiaries as possible.[14]

- Even if plans are relatively subtle about dissuading sick beneficiaries from enrolling, or encouraging the sick to disenroll, there is the chance that HCFA or the press may find out, and the threat of bad publicity or sanctions is serious.

- If a plan does not include in its network hospitals with good reputations, it may have trouble attracting the healthy as well as the sick.

- If a plan consistently makes it hard for beneficiaries to obtain needed care, and beneficiaries are aware of this, then it will have a hard time persuading both the healthy and the sick to enroll. While those in need may be even less likely than the relatively healthy to enroll—leading to a favorable selection—if overall enrollment is low, a plan will not do well even with favorable selection.

- The culture of a successful organization is one that does a good job of serving its customers. It may be hard to run a well-functioning medical group or HMO if there is a counter-current in the organization that doing an excellent job of serving those most in need is not part of the organization's mission.

- Concerns about medical liability require HMOs to provide services that are "medically necessary" (defined by a community standard of care).

- Most physicians, providers, and health plan administrators are professionals who want to do a good job of taking care of people.

Each of these factors will act as a partial restraint against the financial incentives to HMOs to try to enroll a favorable selection of risks. In the current environment, however, the restraining influences are not enough to fully overcome the financial incentives. HCFA's task is to increase the power of the restraining influences.

RISK SELECTION IN MATURE MEDICARE MARKETS

The extent to which favorable selection is likely to persist in more mature HMO markets is uncertain, but it seems likely that even in relatively mature markets HMOs will receive a favorable selection of Medicare beneficiaries under current HCFA policy. Two factors reduce selection effects in markets in which HMO penetration is higher and in which larger numbers of beneficiaries have been enrolled for longer periods of time. First, beneficiaries who enroll in HMOs when they have particularly low utilization will have their expected healthcare needs increase over time.[15] Second, when larger numbers of beneficiaries have enrolled in plans, if some enrollees with heavy care needs are well served in HMOs, word of this is likely to spread, and those with heavy care needs may be more likely to enroll than when penetration is low. However, even at 40 percent or 50 percent or 60 percent HMO penetration it is likely, under current rules, that there would still be substantial differences in health status between HMO enrollees and beneficiaries in fee-for-service: greater consumer preferences for HMOs among the healthy than among the sick, as well as the financial imperative for plans to avoid an adverse risk mix combined with ample opportunity for taking actions to influence enrollment composition suggest a continuation of favorable selection even in mature markets. Recent General Accounting Office testimony on the extent of risk selection in high penetration counties in California provides some support for this expectation, although it should be noted that even in the counties with high penetration most of the HMO enrollment is quite recent (USGAO 1997).

NOTES

1. Useful articles that review the Medicare risk selection literature are: Rossiter et al. 1989, Davidson et al. 1992, Helliger 1987, and Riley et al. 1996. Numerous others that report analytic results are referenced below.
2. Bryan Dowd, personal communication, 2/25/98, notes that a study recently completed for HCFA found that people enrolled in an HMO in April 1993 were about 50 percent less likely to die in the subsequent two years than people who were in fee-for-service on that date, controlling for numerous factors, including the AAPCC payment cells, payment rates, county mortality rates, and HMO penetration rates and enrollment growth rates. (The study sample size for HMO enrollees was about 1.5 million, 21,000 disenrollees, and 1.2 million beneficiaries in fee-for-service.) Some earlier work found some HMOs where mortality rates were inconsistent with other indicators of selection bias. For example, Langwell and Hadley (1989) mention one HMO whose Medicare enrollees had higher prior reimbursements but lower mortality than comparable fee-for-service beneficiaries. However, this HMO's enrollees had high service utilization while in the HMO, suggesting that mortality rates were not an accurate reflection of biased selection in this case. See also Kasper et al. 1988 and Porell and Turner 1990.
3. Approximately 5 percent of Medicare beneficiaries die each year, and last-year-of-life care for these decedents accounts for approximately 28 percent of total Medicare expenditures (Riley, Lubitz, and Rabey 1991 and

Langwell and Hadley 1989). Thus, decedents have a weight of 5.6 and survivors have a weight of 0.758. In fee-for-service, the overall weight is $(0.05 \times 5.6) + (.95 \times .758) = 1.0$. If the HMO mortality rate is 25 percent lower, then the HMO overall weight is $(0.0375 \times 5.6) + (.9625 \times .758) =$ .943. While in theory lower mortality rates among HMO enrollees may be endogenous, resulting from higher quality care, in practice it seems likely that almost all of the observed difference in mortality between HMO and fee-for-service beneficiaries is a result of selection effects.

4. The best study arguing against the consensus on favorable persistent risk selection is by Rodgers and Smith (1996), commissioned by the American Association of Health Plans.

5. The Center for Studying Health System Change (1996) notes that the sample is very small—only 371 HMO enrollees; is not designed to be representative of HMO risk contract enrollees; and could be biased because it excludes people who died during the first nine months of the study period and does not capture the effects of switching between HMOs and fee-for-service. A CBO memorandum (July 17, 1996) is cited that argues that adjusting for these biases could more than quadruple the estimate of favorable selection in the Rodgers and Smith study.

6. J. Dubow in *Improving the Medicare Market* (1996) provides a good recent literature review. She cites the following studies of Medicare beneficiaries: Clement et al. (1994) found no significant outcome differences for Medicare HMO and FFS beneficiaries with chest pain or joint pain on three of four measures, the exception being that HMO enrollees had less symptomatic improvement of joint pain. Carlisle et al. (1992) found no mortality differences for HMO and Medicare fee-for-service patients who had been hospitalized with acute myocardial infarction.

7. Two other advantages of joining an HMO—better coordination of care and reduced paperwork—do increase as people get sicker, but they are minor compared with the monetary incentive. These were not mentioned among the most commonly cited reasons for joining plans in a recent survey of enrollees (Nelson et al. 1996), although the reduced burden of paperwork has been mentioned by respondents in other surveys cited by Dubow (1996).

8. Analysis of the Medicare Current Beneficiary Survey shows that 11 percent of the community aged elderly do not have either Medicaid or private supplemental coverage (Chulis et al. 1995); however, the Current Population Survey finds 22 percent without supplemental coverage (Ways and Means Committee, Green Book), and the National Health Interview Survey finds 25 percent without supplemental coverage (Congressional Budget Office 1997). We do not know why the CBS results are so different from the CPS and NHIS results.

9. In the CBS data, approximately one-third of low-income beneficiaries do not have supplemental coverage; for these beneficiaries in particular, those who are sick may be more attracted to HMOs than those who are healthy.

10. Only 4 percent of the Medicare disabled are enrolled in HMOs, compared to 12 percent of the over-65 beneficiaries. Given that approximately 50 percent

of Medicare disabled also have Medicaid, perhaps a fairer comparison is among the disabled without Medicaid. Even so, 8 percent penetration is well under the overall Medicare average. Because the AAPCC adjusts for disability status, this is not in itself evidence of favorable selection (remember that selection is defined relative to the group upon which capitation rates are based).

11. The GAO conducted a similar exercise in 1996. They received information from only 10 of 14 HMOs even after follow-up calls. Graphic pictures are included in the report showing an 8-inch stack of documents from the HMOs, which cover an entire wall, distilled into a 3-page side-by-side benefit comparison sheet compiled by HCFA.

12. Institute of Medicine (1996) reports research results on Medicare beneficiary information needs, both content and form.

13. The influence of provider networks can be seen in Tollen and Rothman (1998), which shows that an HMO in Colorado serving Medicaid patients, which had contracted with a University hospital and a children's hospital, had a massively adverse selection of patients.

14. Merlis et al. (1998) provide a good discussion of the tension between plan marketers and actuaries.

15. This "regression towards the mean" effect has been discussed by Welch (1985). An individual with expected annual expenditures of $2,500 is more likely to enroll in an HMO following a good year, in which actual expenditures were only $1,000, than following a bad year with expenditures of $5,000 (because of the attachment to physicians arguments made above). The individual's expected expenditures in the first year following enrollment may be $1,800 but a few years later it will be $2,500. The extent of favorable selection decreases over time. However, if the individuals who do enroll are inherently healthier than those who do not, even after many years of enrollment, health status differences will remain between the two groups: individuals regress toward their own mean, not toward the mean of a demographically defined group.

REFERENCES

Adams, M., and J. Tyler. 1995. "Medicare Risk HMO Performance Indicators" (abstract). *Association for Health Services Research Annual Meeting Abstract Book* 12 (37).

Berki, S., and M. Ashcroft. 1980. "HMO Enrollment: Who Joins What and Why? A Review of the Literature." *Milbank Memorial Fund Quarterly* 58 (4): 588–642.

Billi, J., C. Wise, S. Sher, L. Duran-Arenas, and L. Shapiro. 1993. "Selection in a Preferred Provider Organization Enrollment." *Health Services Research* 28 (5): 563–75.

Brown, R., J. Bergeron, D. Clement, J. Hill, and S. Retchin. 1993. "The Medicare Risk Program for HMOs—Final Summary Report on Findings from the Evaluation." Report submitted to the Department of Health and Human Services. Princeton, NJ: Mathematica Policy Research, Inc.

Center for Studying Health System Change. 1996. "Policy Implications of Risk Selection in Medicare HMOs, Is the Federal Payment Rate Too High?" Issues Brief no 4.

Chulis, G. S., F. J. Epping, M. O. Hogan, D. R. Waldo, and R. H. Arnett III. 1995. "Health Insurance and the Elderly: Data from the MCBS." *Health Care Financing Review* 14 (3): 163–81.

Congressional Budget Office. 1997. *Predicting How Changes in Medicare's Payment Rates Would Affect Risk-Sector Enrollment and Costs.* Washington, DC.

Dallek, G., A. Harper, C. Jimenez, and C. Daw. 1993. "Medicare Risk Contracting HMOs in California: A Study of Marketing, Quality and Due Process Rights." Los Angeles: Center for Health Care Rights.

Davidson, B. N., S. Sofaer, and P. Gertler. 1992. "Consumer Information and Biased Selection in the Demand for Coverage Medicare." *Social Science and Medicine* 34 (9): 1023–34.

Dowd, B., R. Feldman, I. Moscovice, C. Wisner, P. Bland, and M. Finch. 1996. "An Analysis of Selectivity Bias in the Medicare AAPCC." *Health Care Financing Review* 17 (3): 35–57.

Dowd, B., I. Moscovice, R. Feldman, M. Finch, C. Wisner, and S. Hillson. 1994. "Health Plan Choice in the Twin Cities Medicare Market." *Medical Care* 32 (10): 1019–39.

Dubow, J. 1996. "Medicare Managed Care: Issues for Vulnerable Populations." In *Improving the Medicare Market.* Washington, DC: Institute of Medicine, National Academy Press.

Eggers, P., and R. Prihoda. 1982. "Risk Differential Between Medicare Beneficiaries Enrolled and Not Enrolled in an HMO." *Health Care Financing Review* 4 (1): 55–73.

Garfinkel, S., W. Schlenger, K. McLeroy, F. A. Bryan, B. J. G. York, G. H. Dunteman, and A. S. Friedlob. 1986. "Choice of Payment Plan in the Medicare Capitation Demonstration." *Medical Care* 24 (7): 628–40.

Helliger, F. J. 1987. "Selection Bias in Health Maintenance Organizations: Analysis of Recent Evidence." *Health Care Financing Review* 9 (2): 55–63.

Institute of Medicine. 1996. *Improving the Medicare Market.* Washington, DC: National Academy Press.

Kasper, J., G. Riley, J. McCombs, and M. A. Stevenson. 1988. "Beneficiary Selection, Use and Charges in Two Medicare Capitation Demonstrations." *Health Care Financing Review* 10 (1): 37–49.

Kertesz, L. 1995. "Enrollment, Access Woes Cited at Some Medicare Risk HMOs." *Modern Healthcare* 25 (12): 6.

Komisar, H. L., J. Hunt-McCool, and J. Feder. 1997/98. "Medicare Spending for Elderly Beneficiaries Who Need Long-Term Care." *Inquiry* 34 (4): 302–10.

Langwell, K., and J. Hadley. 1989. "Evaluation of the Medicare Competition Demonstrations." *Health Care Financing Review* 11 (2): 65–80.

Lichtenstein R., J. Thomas, J. Adams-Watson, J. Lepkowski, and B. Simone. 1991. "Selection Bias in TEFRA At-Risk HMOs." *Medical Care* 29 (4): 318–31.

Lichtenstein, R., J. Thomas, B. Watkins, C. Puto, J. Lepkowski, J. Adams-Watson, B. Simone, and D. Vest. 1992. "HMO Marketing and Selection Bias: Are TEFRA HMOs Skimming?" *Medical Care* 30 (4): 329–46.

Maurer, W. 1990. "Medical Underwriting: Staying Ahead of the Competition." *Group Practice Journal* 39 (2): 53.

Nelson, L., M. Gold, R. Brown, A. Ciemnecki, A. Aizer, and K. CyBulski. 1996. *Access to Care in Medicare Managed Care: Results from a 1996 Survey of Enrollees and*

Disenrollees. Washington, DC: Physician Payment Review Commission and Mathematica Policy Research.

Newhouse, J. 1994. "Patients at Risk: Health Reform and Risk Adjustment." *Health Affairs* 13 (1): 132–46.

Physician Payment Review Commission (PPRC). 1996. *Annual Report to Congress 1996.* Washington, DC.

Porell, F., and W. Turner. 1990. "Biased Selection Under an Experimental Enrollment and Marketing Medicare HMO Broker." *Medical Care* 28 (7): 604–15.

Potosky, A., R. Merrill, G. Riley, S. Taplin, W. Barlow, and B. Fireman. 1997. "Breast Cancer Survival and Treatment in Health Maintenance Organization and Fee-for-Service Settings." *Journal of the National Cancer Institute* 89 (22) 1683–91.

Retchin, S. M., R. S. Brown, S. J. Yeh, D. Chu, and L. Moreno. 1997. "Outcomes of Stroke Patients in Medicare Fee for Service and Managed Care." *Journal of the American Medical Association* 278 (2):119–24.

Riley, G., E. Rabey, and J. Kasper. 1989. "Biased Selection and Regression Toward the Mean in Three Medicare HMO Demonstrations: A Survival Analysis of Enrollees and Disenrollees." *Medical Care* 27 (4): 337–51.

Riley, G., J. Lubitz, and E. Rabey. 1991. "Enrollee Health Status Under Medicare Risk Contracts: An Analysis of Mortality Rates." *Health Services Research* 26 (2): 137–63.

Riley, G., C. Tudor, Y. Chiang, and M. Ingber. 1996. "Health Status of Medicare Enrollees in HMOs and Fee-for-Service in 1994." *Health Care Financing Review* 17 (4): 65–73.

Rodgers, J., and K. Smith. 1996. "Is There Biased Selection in Medicare HMOs?" Prepared for the American Association of Health Plans by Health Policy Economics Group. Washington, DC: Price Waterhouse.

Rossiter, L., K. Langwell, T. Wan, and M. Rivnyak. 1989. "Patient Satisfaction Among Elderly Enrollees and Disenrollees in Medicare HMOs, Results from the National Medicare Competition Evaluation." *American Medical Association Journal* 262 (1): 57–63.

Shaugnessey, P., R. Schlenker, and D. Hittle. 1994. "Home Health Care Outcomes Under Capitated and Fee-for-Service Payment." *Health Care Financing Review* 16 (1): 187–221.

Tollen, L., and M. Rothman. 1998. "Colorado Medicaid HMO Risk Adjustment, A Case Study." Draft paper for Conference. *Health-Based Payment: What Do We Know About Risk Adjustment?* Robert Wood Johnson Alpha Center, January 29, 1998.

Tucker, A., and K. Langwell. 1988. "Disenrollment Patterns in Medicare HMOs: A Preliminary Analysis." *Group Health Association of America Journal* 9 (1): 22–41.

United States General Accounting Office (USGAO). 1986. *Issues Raised by Florida Health Maintenance Organization Demonstrations.* Washington, DC. GAO/HRD-86-07.

United States General Accounting Office. 1997. *Medicare HMOs: HCFA Could Promptly Reduce Excess Payments by Improving Accuracy of County Payment Rates.* Statement of William J. Scanlon, Director Health Financing and Systems, Health, Education and Human Services Division, testimony before the Subcommittee on Health, Committee on Ways and Means, House of Representatives. GAO/HEHS-97-78.

United States General Accounting Office. 1996. *Medicare: HCFA Should Release Data to Aid Consumers, Prompt Better HMO Performance.* GAO/HEHS-97-23.

Ware, J., M. Bayliss, W. Rogers, M. Kosinski, and A. Tarlov. 1996. "Differences in 4-Year Health Outcomes for Elderly and Poor, Chronically Ill Patients Treated in HMO and Fee-for-Service Systems: Results from the Medical Outcomes Study." *Journal of the American Medical Association* 276 (13): 1039–47.

Welch, W. 1985. "Medicare Capitation Payments to HMOs in Light of Regression Towards the Mean in Health Care Costs." In *Advances in Health Economics and Health Services Research*, edited by R. Scheffler and L. Rossiter, 75–96. Greenwich CT: JAI Press Inc.

Paying Plans to Care for People with Chronic Illness

Tony Dreyfus and Richard Kronick

As enrollment of Medicare beneficiaries in health plans continues to climb, more attention is focused on how these health plans are paid. While each of the strategies explored in subsequent chapters can help Medicare buy better services for its beneficiaries and reduce risk selection, financing does much to determine the market environment in which the other strategies will operate. Among various strategies available to Medicare, health-based payment is key.

After a long period of technical development and advocacy among health policy circles, health-based payment is finally being implemented already by a few state Medicaid programs and commercial payors and soon by Medicare. Through the Balanced Budget Act of 1997, Congress directed HCFA to begin health-based payment for Medicare beneficiaries enrolled in health plans in 2000.

Health-based payment is a system of capitated reimbursement that varies payments according to health status. Health-based payment can vary payments to reflect the predictable needs of health plan members far better than traditional risk adjustment based on demographic information.

If payments are not adjusted for health status, Medicare makes wasteful overpayments and various measures to promote quality run against the strong current created by the financing system. The overpayments can be large in a system like Medicare, where managed care enrollment is voluntary.

Without health-based payment, plans can profit much more easily by enrolling low-risk beneficiaries than by competing on quality, because unadjusted rates penalize quality that attracts beneficiaries with above-average needs.

If rates vary with health status, enrollment of high-risk members is rewarded by higher payments, and other Medicare strategies to promote quality will work in tandem with the financial incentives instead of against them. Adjustment by health status will sharply reduce the chronic overpayments to plans with favorable selections of beneficiaries.

The first section of this chapter explains why health-based payment is crucial to cost-effectiveness, fairness, and quality of capitated managed care. The second section outlines various approaches to health-based payment, and the third section describes some of the challenges of the leading method, which uses diagnoses. The fourth section examines how past payment methods and the changes mandated by the Balanced Budget Act will affect the operation and reception of health-based payment. The final two sections describe what is known about HCFA's plans and options in implementation.

USING PAYMENT TO SUPPORT COST-EFFECTIVENESS, FAIRNESS, AND QUALITY

Like a commercial buyer of health coverage, Medicare pays most health plans with capitated payments—a set monthly amount for each beneficiary's coverage regardless of how much health service is actually provided. The capitated payment gives plans the power and resources to bargain, to coordinate care, and to innovate. Because health plans can keep the difference between the capitation and their costs, capitated financing also rewards plans that provide services efficiently. Yet capitated payments can also lead to unnecessary overpayments, can encourage plans to skimp on services, and can discourage them from developing a high level of quality.

Overpayments

Hopes that managed care can be used to contain Medicare costs and assure quality are threatened by the lack of health-based rates. Because enrollment in managed care for Medicare beneficiaries is voluntary, paying rates unadjusted by health status usually leads to wasteful overpayments. People with greater healthcare needs tend to stay in fee-for-service, while managed care plans attract a healthier enrollment. By not adjusting for health status, Medicare overpays plans and still must pay the higher bills of the adverse selection remaining in fee-for-service (PPRC 1996).

In addition, if capitation rates continue to be based on the less healthy beneficiaries in fee-for-service, the overpayment is aggravated (PPRC 1997).

The overpayments get worse, because the movement of healthier beneficiaries into managed care leaves a more costly group in fee-for-service on whom future rates are based.

Fairness

The fairness of payment can be viewed in two ways: fairness among health plans and fairness among beneficiaries. Unfairness arises among plans when the occasional plan that attracts beneficiaries with above-average healthcare needs is paid roughly the same per member as a typical plan that enrolls a favorable selection. Plans that attract people with greater needs should not be penalized with financial losses while plans with a less needy population enjoy undeserved profits.

Unfairness among beneficiaries arises over time as healthier beneficiaries join managed care plans and enjoy supplemental benefits not available to those who stay in fee-for-service arrangements. Medicare rules and competition for beneficiaries push plans to use surpluses for reducing premiums and providing supplemental benefits. Plans that enjoy more substantial favorable selection can afford greater reductions in premium and more extensive supplemental benefits.

This system has the advantage of directing a portion of the overpayments toward Medicare beneficiaries in the form of supplemental benefits. But this use of overpayments unfairly channels saving toward those types of beneficiaries most attracted to health plans and offers no benefit to those, particularly less healthy beneficiaries, who have stayed in fee-for-service arrangements.

Quality

With average rates that do not reflect the health status of actual members, plans that excel in quality and attract a growing number of people with above-average needs find that their successes in improving quality lead to financial losses. Making capitated payments that reflect health status is therefore an essential part of efforts to improve managed care quality.

As described in other chapters, payors can take a variety of steps to make health plans more attentive to quality, but health-based payment is one of the key tools (Enthoven 1988). Even when payors insist on a set of rules to structure the market, plans retain control over their provider networks—which greatly influences a consumer's choice of plan. Nor can monitoring motivate plans to devote themselves energetically to improving quality for those with above-average levels of need, because the enrollment of these individuals leads to losses in a system of average payments.

Health-based payment plays a more ambitious role in the payor's effort to maximize value. The goal of health-based payment is to set rates so that plans compete on quality and get paid more by attracting people with greater needs. When beneficiaries with greater needs can choose among plans that are competing for their enrollment, positive models of managed care will be encouraged.

A positive model of managed care would build itself around the needs of people with disability or chronic illness—coordinating the variety of needed services, providing care to prevent complications, directing people promptly to needed specialists, and providing medical advice and attention around the clock and in people's neighborhoods and homes as an alternative to hospitalization. Such plans would provide up-to-date information and access to new therapies and would continue to care for people even in advanced stages of illness. By contrast, negative models of managed care would fail to coordinate services, miss opportunities for prevention, delay or limit access to needed specialists, and offer impersonal emergency room care outside of business hours and few options for care outside the hospital. People toward the end of their lives would find plans reluctant to provide the needed high levels of medical and supportive care.

Capitation offers the flexibility that plans need to innovate, to develop responsive systems, and to invest in prevention. But if capitated payments are not health-based, then the easiest way to make money is to avoid developing quality that will attract those with greater needs. Average rates give incentives that are precisely opposite of the ideal: a reward of profits for doing the wrong thing and a penalty of losses for doing the right thing. The purpose of health-based payment is to fundamentally reverse the incentives created by the payment system: pay substantially more to plans that attract and serve those with greater needs and pay less to plans that do not. A far higher level of quality should result if beneficiaries with greater needs are choosing among health plans that truly want to serve them.

The benefits of health-based payment are larger for populations with a greater degree of predictability in their healthcare needs. If almost all of a population's healthcare expenditures are unpredictable, then plans can do little to attract or avoid members with greater than average needs. And if needs are almost entirely unpredictable, then no system of health-based payment could be used or would need to be used to adjust payments.

Conversely, if chronic, ongoing needs cause a substantial proportion of the expenditures, then plans will know that their decisions about network, quality, and style can attract a membership with costs predictably greater than or less than average. Fortunately, under such circumstances, the payor can also create a system of payments that vary according to predictable needs, so that plans are appropriately paid.

As we have argued elsewhere, the need and potential for health-based payment appear greatest among Medicaid beneficiaries with disability, for whom expenditures are quite predictable (Kronick et al. 1996). The need and potential for health-based payment among Medicare beneficiaries are somewhat less but are far greater than for commercially insured populations. Medicare beneficiaries with fairly predictable costs include five million individuals under age 65 covered because of significant disability and a large proportion of the almost 34 million Medicare beneficiaries age 65 or over, many of whom experience some chronic illness or ongoing healthcare needs.

The greater ongoing needs for healthcare among these Medicare beneficiaries accentuate both the importance of quality and the disadvantage of average rates. Compared with a general population, costs for people with disabilities or chronic illness are much more predictable: from year to year, high-cost people are likely to stay high-cost, and low-cost individuals are likely to stay low-cost. With average rates, a plan knows very well that if its quality attracts too many people who already have costly chronic conditions it will lose money now and in the future.

Plans may understandably choose not to contract with hospitals, physicians, and other providers who serve many people with serious chronic illness or disability because the reputations and established patient relationships of such specialized providers are likely to attract members with above-average needs. Because the bulk of healthcare expenditures are made for the small proportion of people with substantial needs, a quality advantage that attracts only a small additional number of people with high costs can cause substantial losses. Individuals with conditions such as kidney disease, hemophilia, quadriplegia, or serious cancers and heart diseases are obviously likely to need expensive services. Conversely, a plan that can avoid its fair share of people with greater needs can greatly reduce its costs.

How Good Do Predictions Need to Be?

Advocates of managed care have argued since the 1970s that effective health-based payment or risk adjustment would greatly help shift the attention of health plans away from strategies for avoiding sick people and toward strategies for improving quality. It would be hard to find a healthcare economist or policy analyst to disagree.

But health plans have expressed doubts about moving forward to implementation and have questioned whether recently developed systems are adequate to the task. Some opposition has come from health plans understandably concerned that they will have to make new investments in information systems and that their profitable Medicare payments will be reduced. Among disinterested observers, doubt has arisen in part from appropriate concerns and in part from some misunderstandings about health-based payment.

One misconception is that highly accurate predictions of individual expenditures are possible and needed. In fact, *no* method will ever predict healthcare costs for individuals very accurately because most healthcare is provided in response to unpredictable needs. Precisely which individuals will experience an accident, pneumonia, or a serious cancer, for example, cannot be known in advance. Even for groups with serious chronic conditions and related predictable costs, much of the variation in individual costs cannot be predicted by any method.

Fortunately, no payment system needs to predict the unpredictable. As both an arranger of services and an insurer, each health plan covers unpredictable variation in individual costs using the capitation received for all members to pay for the few members who need extensive care. And plans protect against the chance that unpredictable needs will exceed their income through financial reserves or reinsurance. The goal of health-based payment is not to compensate plans for the *unpredictable*, insured risk but to pay for the *predictable* risk, so that plans will gladly serve individuals with predictably higher needs. For example, it is important to pay plans correctly on average for people with serious renal disease, but it is not necessary to pay even more for those individuals with renal disease who this year have unpredictable complications.

Plans can always use their knowledge of individual members, especially their recent healthcare expenditures, to identify individuals who likely will cost more or less than what the payment system provides for them. As a result, health-based payment must be part of a larger strategy by which the payor guides plans to focus on quality instead of selectively avoiding beneficiaries who are less profitable to serve.

Yet payors should not be too discouraged that plans will usually know their members better than the payor does. Getting the payments close to right can do much to set the incentives that will motivate plans to pursue quality. With traditional rates set at average costs for a large group of eligible beneficiaries, all the members on whom a plan consistently loses money are obviously those with serious chronic needs while all the "profitable" members are those with below-average needs. Plans are powerfully discouraged by predictable losses from developing quality that will attract individuals with chronic conditions and powerfully encouraged by predictable profits to attract people with below-average needs. The carrot and the stick are large and obvious, both pointing in the wrong direction—away from quality for people with greater needs.

In contrast, even though the health-based capitation does not perfectly reflect the predictable needs of each individual, the "money-losing" members and the "profitable" members are scattered across all levels of need. With appropriate payments to cover members with serious chronic conditions, health plans find that for some people with serious illness the costs of care exceed payments, while for others with serious illness the payments exceed the costs. Similarly, for people without serious chronic illness, plans lose money on some and make money on others. Plans no longer profit easily by avoiding individuals with high levels of need, because a plan that enrolls disproportionately low-risk members will be paid less than average. And a plan that enrolls many with serious illness will receive adequate funds. To survive and prosper, either type of plan will need to focus on improving the quality and cost-effectiveness of care.

APPROACHES TO HEALTH-BASED PAYMENT

A longstanding consensus in health policy circles exists about the importance of health-based payment, but extensive research and debate on *how* health-based payment should be done is more recent. The challenge is to find a practical way to measure beneficiaries' predictable health risk that can be used to vary payments appropriately. Most of the recent research and development of health-based payment systems has focused on using diagnostic information. Some questions about implementation remain, but the basic approach of using diagnoses to adjust payments appears the most promising. Good diagnostic classification systems that payors need to implement health-based payment are now available.

The Demographic Approach

Medicare has long practiced traditional risk adjustment, paying plans different amounts depending on each enrolled beneficiary's demographic characteristics, including age, sex, and county of residence. Different amounts are also paid if the beneficiary has state Medicaid benefits because of low income, is living in a nursing home or other institution, or is a Medicare beneficiary because of disability.

Consider the majority of beneficiaries who are age 65 or over, without Medicaid coverage and not living in institutions. Among such beneficiaries, Medicare pays one rate for all women age 70 to 74 living in Cook County and one somewhat higher rate for women age 75 to 79 in Cook County—about 18 percent higher.[1] This demographic approach has the virtue of using data that is very easy to get and is not subject to manipulation by plans. Unfortunately, traditional demographic rates reflect individuals' health status very poorly. A 75-year-old woman is *on average* likely to need more healthcare than a 70-year-old woman, but if the older woman is healthy and the younger woman has a serious liver disease, then the demographic rates fail completely to reflect their different levels of need.

The essential problem with demographic rates is that any age-gender group in a county will include many people with good health and some with significant chronic illness, and plans can easily attract the healthy and not the sick. Among men age 65 to 69 living in Los Angeles County, for example, many are quite healthy, some have intermediate levels of healthcare needs, and a smaller group of men has very serious chronic illnesses or disability. Those with serious illnesses such as congestive heart failure or liver disease can be expected to have annual costs three to four times more than those with no significant chronic conditions, and those with even more serious problems or multiple chronic conditions can be expected to cost even more.[2] From each demographic rate group, Medicare HMOs have tended to enroll disproportionately healthy people and disproportionately few people with greater needs; as a result, the demographic rates fail to reflect the lower risk they face and lead to systematic overpayments.

A General Mandate to Move to Adjusting Rates by Diagnoses

The BBA introduces a host of changes to the Medicare program, including health-based payment for Medicare managed care, now to be known as the Medicare+Choice program. The BBA mandates that health-based payment begin in 2000 but specifies little about implementation. The BBA requires health plans to begin reporting inpatient diagnoses that can be used for rate adjustment, a provision in effect from the beginning of 1998. The act also authorizes the collection of ambulatory data, which many plans find harder to report, as early as July 1998 if deemed necessary by the Secretary of Health and Human Services. (We take up a variety of issues raised by the BBA in the following sections.)

In the bigger picture of the development of risk adjustment, the BBA marks a critical turning point: the largest payor has decided to begin health-based payment and to do so using diagnoses. For a variety of reasons, diagnoses currently appear to be the most practical and effective kind of data to use. Diagnoses are directly related to healthcare need and allow good predictions of future expenditures. Practical considerations about implementation also support the use of diagnoses, which are routinely collected, are available in Medicare and Medicaid claims, and can be audited. Research groups have developed several good diagnostic classification systems that Medicare and other payors can use to implement health-based payment.

Other Kinds of Data

But use of other kinds of data will continue to receive attention over the next few years and may soon be used to supplement or even replace the use of diagnostic data.

The *functional status approach* uses data on an individual's degree of disability as measured by ability to perform activities such as getting out of bed, bathing, dressing, and preparing meals (Gruenberg, Kaganova, and Hornbrook 1996). Data from functional assessments can play an important role in making payments for nursing home or other long-term care and may one day help in rate setting for acute healthcare. But functional status data are not yet available for the large populations required in setting rates for healthcare.

Surveys could help supply the information, but their substantial costs per person would mean that information would be gathered on only a sample of beneficiaries in each plan. Sampling of beneficiaries who remain in fee-for-service would also be needed to estimate the differences in health status between plan members and average beneficiaries. Alternatively, the government could require plans to perform periodic functional assessments of Medicare beneficiaries and to report it along with other required data such as diagnoses.

Self-reported or *independent assessment* of health status currently faces the same limitations as functional data. Self-reported assessment means asking beneficiaries about their health status, and could include questions about specific diagnoses, functional status, or overall health. The required surveys would be fairly costly, and the level of detail of the diagnostic information would be far less than what is available from clinical data.

Independent assessment of health status (e.g., as used currently for disability determination) would be fairly costly, but it would have the significant advantage of not being subject to manipulation by health plans. Independent assessment could include diagnostic, functional, and self-reported assessment of health status.

If there is ever any movement toward payments based on *outcomes*, then independent assessment may become especially valuable. If plans are to be paid based on their performance in improving or maintaining the health status of their members, independent assessment of members' health status would be much more important.

The use of outcome measures would seem to avoid a potential problem of diagnostic-based payment—that payment will fall when a plan member no longer experiences a chronic condition, apparently creating an incentive to keep people sick. We think this incentive problem is not too real, at least for prospective payment: curing a chronic illness brings a boosted payment next year *and* avoids the costs of the ongoing illness. By identifying but not treating an illness, the plan would get a higher payment next year but would also face an ongoing risk of higher costs, not to mention sanctions for failure to treat.

In addition, establishing outcomes measures for rate setting would be very complicated. As long as healthcare is primarily *medicine*—that is, the treatment of problems—we think the diagnoses that describe health problems will continue to be the best predictor of cost and the most appropriate basis for rate setting.

The *prior expenditure approach* uses an individual's past healthcare expenditures, which predict future needs quite accurately. For example, Medicare could set a capitation payment for a plan's members based on their recent fee-for-service bills, which would be easy for beneficiaries moving from fee-for-service into managed care.

Adjustment by prior expenditures alone could not be sustained for long, however, without a substantial shift in policy and contracting practices. In time, fee-for-service data will be out of date for older enrollees, and many newer enrollees may have no prior fee-for-service data. To continue adjusting by prior expenditures, Medicare could switch from adjusting by prior fee-for-service data to adjusting by expenditures that the plans make for their own enrollees. But now, the more plans spend on their enrollees in any year, the more they would be paid in the following year. One of capitation's basic goals—to encourage efficient provision of care—would be largely undermined as the incentives created by the payment system would revert to those of fee-for-service, with a one-year lag (Kronick and Dreyfus 1997).

Prior Expenditure, Risk Sharing, and Partial Capitation

The use of prior expenditure data to vary payments is closely related to two financing options: risk sharing and partial capitation. In all these arrangements, payment partly depends on how much services are delivered, which lessens both the good and bad incentives of full-risk capitation—positively, to provide services efficiently and, negatively, to underserve members. In a risk-sharing arrangement, the payor and plan may agree, for example, that the plan will assume the risk (profit or loss) if medical expenses turn out to be anywhere from 5 percent below to 5 percent above the capitation, but that the next 10 percent of savings or loss will be split 50–50, and that beyond 15 percent, most or all risk will be assumed by the payor.

Risk sharing is mathematically equivalent to a proposal for partial capitation, which would mix capitation with fee-for-service payments to strike a balance between their respective incentives to underserve and to provide too much care (Newhouse, Buntin, and Chapman 1997). A 50–50 blend of capitation and fee-for-service, for example, is financially identical to full capitation with risk of profits or losses shared 50–50 between payor and plan. In both cases, a plan considering whether a member needs an additional service knows that half of the expenditure will be covered by the payor. One difference between risk sharing and partial capitation is that risk-sharing arrangements can be structured so that the plan is responsible for most or all risk if expenditures are close to the total capitation payments, with the payor assuming a greater proportion of risk only when expenditures and total capitation payments differ substantially.

The arguments for risk sharing and partial capitation, however, have been based on some different assumptions about plans' cost structures, leading to different expectations about resulting incentives. Risk sharing appears only to *reduce* the incentive for the plan to avoid a beneficiary whose costs are expected to exceed the health-based payment. The plan still views such a beneficiary as a money-losing member whom the plan would be better off without. If we assume, however, as Newhouse does in his argument for partial capitation, that the marginal cost of services is less than the average cost, then risk sharing appears more helpful. With the assumption of lower marginal costs, the plan would appear perfectly happy to provide additional services because it knows that the additional cost will be covered by the risk-sharing arrangement.

The argument for partial capitation, as made by Newhouse, builds on Pauly's notion of an ideal price for insured health services, which is set where the additional cost of providing the service is equal to the value perceived by an informed consumer (Pauly 1980). A payor could aim for the ideal price by a payment that blends—say 50–50 or 60–40—capitation and fee-for-service payments. The half or partial capitation would help cover ongoing expenses, while the half or partial fees for services would cover the marginal cost of services provided, leaving the plan indifferent as to whether to provide more or less service. Partial capitation would thus compromise correctly between the extreme of fee-for-service, in which the provider is encouraged to provide too much service, and full capitation, where the plan is encouraged to provide too little. Because rate setters do not know plans' marginal costs, establishing the ideal blend of capitation and fee-for-service could be a matter for experimentation (Newhouse, Buntin, and Chapman 1997).

Risk sharing and partial capitation share some of the disadvantages of capitation based on prior expenditures. The payor and plan must define the types and rates of expenditures for which risk will be shared, and a detailed settlement is required. The flexibility of plans to substitute new services may be compromised. And plans may find that Medicare is unwilling to recognize plans' actual administrative costs, which are typically much higher than those incurred by a payor of fee-for-service bills.

Risk sharing or partial capitation still appear to be good concepts, but their difficulties suggest that Medicare should place more priority on implementing health-based payment and see later whether risk sharing is possible. Implementation of health-based payment is moving forward, and it would be unwise to let the difficulties of risk sharing hold up progress in health-based payment. Once health-based payment is more widely implemented, some larger experiments with risk sharing or partial capitation would be valuable.[3] The BBA provisions allowing for reinsurance and risk sharing may let HCFA offer arrangements fairly similar in effect to partial capitation. HCFA would then have an excellent opportunity to learn how plans will respond to such arrangements and how difficult their administration proves to be.

Adjusting for Provision of End-of-Life Care

Adjusting payments for provision of end-of-life care is a promising approach that has so far received little public discussion. Paying more to plans that care for a disproportionate share of beneficiaries in their final year of life would provide needed resources to these plans and encourage plans to provide attentive care even to members that are failing. And almost 30 percent of Medicare expenditures are made for the 5 percent of beneficiaries who are in their final year of life (Lubitz and Riley 1993). Policymakers have shied from the possibility of paying more for end-of-life care because of the negative appearance that they would be "paying for death." But the virtues of this approach in its simplicity and in providing incentives to improve end-of-life care merit further attention. The final section of this chapter offers more discussion.

THE CHALLENGE OF DIAGNOSTIC ADJUSTMENT: MOVING TO FULL REPORTS

Health-based payment for Medicare plans will initially be based only on the most serious principal diagnosis made during beneficiaries' inpatient hospital stays. HCFA plans to use the Principal Inpatient Diagnostic Cost Group (PIPDCG) model developed by Arlene Ash, Randy Ellis, Greg Pope, and colleagues based on analysis of expenditures for a large sample of Medicare beneficiaries (Ellis et al. 1996). This appears to be the right approach, but, as we argue in this section, it is not the right approach to stick with for too long. Full diagnostic reports are needed for health-based payment to work on an ongoing basis.

Initial Virtues of Adjustment by Inpatient Diagnoses Only

Adjustment by principal inpatient diagnoses only will be relatively easy, because only a single piece of new information will be required beyond the traditional demographics used for rate setting. The diagnostic data will be reported for only the minority of Medicare beneficiaries who are hospitalized during a given year—about one-fifth (Ellis et al. 1996a, 106). Hospitals are accustomed to reporting these inpatient diagnoses, which have for many years been a part of Medicare's hospital payment system. By contrast, some plans will face significant challenges in gathering ambulatory diagnoses, which are made for a majority of beneficiaries in a wide variety of settings.

Using only the single most serious inpatient diagnosis also would have the advantage of making the payment system less subject to gaming. Plans could not boost their estimated level of risk simply by adding more diagnoses to a member's record, and Medicare could more stringently audit a single diagnosis than it could multiple diagnoses.

Compared to the demographic approach, adjusting payments based on principal inpatient diagnoses does much to improve the accuracy of payments, providing more appropriate levels of payment to plans that enroll individuals with chronic needs and less opportunity for profit to plans that enroll a disproportionately healthy membership. The degree of improvement can be seen by taking subgroups selected according to their characteristics in a first year and comparing how much of their costs in the second year are paid for by the demographic or the health-based approach. (As part of evaluation of risk adjustment models, various comparisons are made of such "predictive ratios," the ratio of predicted expenditures that the system would pay to the actual expenditures.)

For example, among the one-fifth of Medicare beneficiaries who were most expensive in 1991, the demographic approach would pay less than half their actual costs in 1992, while payments on demographics and principal inpatient diagnoses would pay 85 percent of actual expenditures. For those with a diagnosis in 1991 hospital or physician claims of diabetes with complications, the demographic approach would pay 45 percent of 1992 expenditures while adjusting by the principal inpatient diagnosis would pay 69 percent (see Table 3.1 below; discussion of the ADDCG and HCC models are farther below).

The Wrong Incentives of Staying with Inpatient Diagnoses Only

Despite the relative ease and the significant effectiveness of implementing health-based payment with inpatient diagnoses only, it would be inadvisable to use this approach on an extended basis. Because adjustments are based on the diagnoses recorded while beneficiaries are enrolled in plans, using inpatient diagnoses only will create a strong incentive for plans to encourage hospitalization of their members. Plans expecting that HCFA will

Table 3.1 Predictive Ratios of Age-Sex, DCG, and HCC Models for Selected Validation Groups

Validation Groups Selected by 1991 Characteristics	Ratios of Predicted 1992 Expenditures to Actual 1992 Expenditures			
	Age-Sex	PIPDCG	ADDCG	HCC
1991 Expenditures				
Lowest cost quintile of beneficiaries	2.49	1.92	1.22	1.30
Second quintile	1.78	1.37	1.37	1.24
Third quintile	1.31	1.01	1.24	1.14
Fourth quintile	.91	.78	1.02	.99
Highest cost quintile	.48	.85	.78	.85
1991 Diagnoses				
Hip fracture	.59	.86	.85	.99
Depression	.58	.81	.80	.87
Heart failure/cardiomyopathy	.48	.74	.87	.98
Diabetes with complications	.45	.69	.81	.93
Lung or pancreas cancer	.32	.64	.89	.92

Source: Ellis, R. P., et al. 1996. "Diagnosis-Based Risk Adjustment for Medicare Capitation Payments." *Health Care Financing Review* 17 (3): 115–16.

move promptly to using all diagnoses are unlikely to shift care into the hospital. But if it appears that the use of hospital data only will continue for a substantial period, this could impede the development of high-quality ambulatory services. The shifting of services from inpatient to ambulatory care has likely been one of the most important means of containing costs without adversely affecting outcomes.

In addition, some plans that have already succeeded in reducing inpatient care may find their payments unfairly reduced. Plans with low PIPDCG case-mix scores will most likely have even lower scores when case mix is evaluated with the greater detail from all diagnoses. But plans that have made special efforts to reduce hospitalization may understandably object to extended use of inpatient-only adjustment.

Some may argue that most of the incremental payments associated with diagnoses in an inpatient-only system are not enough to provide plans with incentives to hospitalize. For example, in the Principal Inpatient Diagnostic Cost Group Model (PIPDCG), the six lowest of the 12 diagnostic cost groups, covering about 90 percent of the beneficiaries, were associated with additional 1992 costs of less than $6,000 (Ellis et al. 1996b).[4] Even projecting such a cost forward to an incremental payment in 2000 of $9,000 or so, one may imagine that it would be hardly worthwhile for a plan to send someone to the hospital.[5] The additional $9,000 payment that would be received the following year if the beneficiary is still a member would not appear to be worth the certain immediate bill for the hospitalization.

We would argue, however, that the incentive problem is still serious, even for these modest PIPDCGs. The choice a plan would often face is not between hospitalizing someone at a cost of $10,000 or not hospitalizing and incurring no costs. The real incentive problem occurs for a beneficiary who is receiving substantial services at home, such as skilled nursing for attention to skin ulcers, intravenous drug therapy for an infection, or mechanical respiratory assistance or cardiac monitoring. Such a person may be doing well at home. Indeed, some of the key innovations that managed care can bring to people with serious chronic illness or disability is to figure out how services that were once seen as deliverable only in the hospital can be brought to people's homes. Sometimes home-based services reduce costs, sometimes they reduce the physical and psychological ill effects of hospitalization, sometimes they do both.

But the home-based services that can substitute for hospitalization are still quite expensive, often costing thousands or even tens of thousands of dollars. The choice that plans face is not between a substantial cost in the hospital and a zero cost at home, but between a substantial cost in the hospital and a substantial cost serving the person with home, community, or outpatient services. If plans are paid large additional amounts only when services are provided and diagnoses made during inpatient stays, it is hard to imagine that they would not be strongly influenced in their decision making by the payment system. It is up to beneficiaries, physicians, and health plans to decide what mix of hospital-based and other services is best; the payment system should not be exerting substantial influence.

The incentive problem also looks serious when we consider some of the more costly diagnostic categories in an inpatient-only system. Some of the PIPDCG categories have fewer numbers of people, but more dollars of increased payment: five with additional associated expenditures of nearly $9,000 to $23,000 in 1992 dollars. For example, PIPDCG 10, with 1992 associated expenditures of $8,931, includes such conditions as manic and depressive disorders, anemia, ventricular tachycardia, and asthma. PIPDCG 12, at $11,248, includes heart failure, diabetes with acute or chronic complications, and hypoglycemia. PIPDCG 14, at $13,728, includes chronic ulcer of skin, emphysema and chronic bronchitis, renal failure, and lung cancer. (See Table 3.2 below for more detail. Before implementation in 2000, the PIPDCG system will be remodeled with more recent, perhaps 1995–1996, data, but the current version should give a very good indication of the general nature of the model that will actually be used.)

If it were the case that almost all people with PIPDCG diagnoses were treated in the hospital, there would be little reason to worry about the system's

Table 3.2 PIPDCG Model with Diagnoses and Annual
Prospective Payment Amounts

PIPDCG	Most Costly Inpatient Diagnosis in 1991 (partial list only for DCGs 10 to 4)	Percentage of Beneficiaries	Additional Cost, 1992
23	Chemotherapy	0.1%	$22,799
17	End-stage liver disorders, respiratory failure or arrest, Hodgkin's disease/lymphoma/ myeloma/leukemia, secondary cancers	0.4	16,952
14	Gastrointestinal cancers, polyneuropathy, chronic skin ulcer, renal failure, emphysema/ chronic bronchitis, lung cancer, lung diseases due to external agents, other lung disease, other blood disease	0.9	13,728
12	Heart failure, diabetes with complications, hypoglycemia, gram-negative/staphylococcus pneumonia, mouth/pharynx/ larynx and other respiratory cancers, arthropathy/bone infection, cancers of placenta/ovary/uterine adnexa	1.7	11,248
10	Septicemia/shock, arterial embolism and thrombosis, manic and depressive disorders, asthma, fluid/electrolyte disorders	2.0	8,931
8	Cerebrovascular disease, rehab procedures, other acute ischemia, peritonitis/intestinal obstruction, colon cancer	4.7	6,886
			Continued

incentives to hospitalize. For a variety of the diagnoses, however, many people with the diagnosis are not hospitalized, many of whom have high expenses for the year. See Table 3.3 below for examples of PIPDCG diagnoses for which substantial numbers of Medicaid beneficiaries with disability have annual costs of more than $12,000 despite having no inpatient claim for the year. For purposes of comparison, we looked at the expenditures for beneficiaries who had certain diagnoses as a principal inpatient diagnosis and those who had them as ambulatory diagnoses while having no inpatient claims for the year. For some diagnoses, such as chemotherapy and end-stage liver disorders, about 95 percent of those with costs of more than $12,000 have been in the hospital, but for many other diagnoses (e.g., manic and depressive disorders or chronic skin ulcer) one-third or more of those with the diagnosis who have costs of more than $12,000 had no hospital stay.[6] The choice of $12,000 as a selection point was arbitrary; of course if this number were lowered to say $6,000 or $9,000, the proportions of individuals with no inpatient stay would be much larger. Data for Medicare beneficiaries over age 65 may differ, but it seems almost certain that for quite a few PIPDCG diagnoses a similar pattern would be found.

Table 3.2   (continued)

PIPDCG	Most Costly Inpatient Diagnosis in 1991 (partial list only for DCGs 10 to 4)	Percentage of Beneficiaries	Additional Cost, 1992
7	Bacterial pneumonia, acute myocardial infarction, dementia, complications of procedures and care, kidney infection	2.1	5,747
6	Femoral fracture, atrial arrythmia, angina, thrombophlebitis, anal/rectal/GI disorders, transient cerebral ischemia	2.5	4,865
5	Back pain, ulcers, cancer of prostate/testis/ male genitals, rhythm and conduction disorders, diverticula of intestine	2.4	4,284
4	Breast cancer, uncomplicated abdominal hernia, osteoarthritis, gall bladder disorders, fracture/dislocation	1.5	3,341
3	Internal/open wound, prostate/testicular/ penile disorders, lower limb fractures, benign neoplasms, ear disorders, skull and face fractures, diseases of female genital organs	0.7	2,651
2	Uncomplicated diabetes, CNS infections, pregnancy/perinatal conditions, genital prolapse, heart arrest/shock, no inpatient claims	80.9	1,859

Note: The model also includes a variable for Medicaid eligiblity and for age-gender categories. Those eligible for Medicaid had additional expenditures of $1,449; the additional expenditures for the age-gender categories ranged from zero for women age 65–69 up to $2,519 for men age 85 older.

Source: Adapted from R. P. Ellis et al. 1996. *Diagnostic Cost Group (DCG) and Hierarchical Coexisting Conditions (HCC) Models for Medicare Risk Adjustment, Final Report.* Waltham, MA: Health Economics Research, Tables 4-2, 4-3, and C-1.

Another important reason to move from basing payments only on inpatient diagnoses to basing payment on inpatient and ambulatory diagnoses is the substantially higher accuracy of payments that can be obtained by using both kinds of diagnoses and paying more for beneficiaries with multiple diagnoses. Using multiple diagnoses to estimate an individual's future needs can yield substantially more accurate rates and thereby provide stronger incentives for plans to enroll people with greater needs.

Accuracy is improved because multiple diagnoses help differentiate someone with a simple illness or disability from someone with a complex condition who has substantially greater healthcare needs. For example, the level of need for someone with congestive heart failure only is on average considerably less than for someone with congestive heart failure *and* diabetes. Someone with uncomplicated paraplegia resulting from cerebral palsy is likely to have much lower costs than someone with paraplegia resulting from spinal cord injury and complicated by substance abuse and decubitus

Table 3.3 Frequency of Disabled Medicaid Beneficiaries with PIPDCG Diagnoses with and without Inpatient Claims and Their Distribution Among Those with Costs Over $12,000

PIPDCG Diagnosis	Number with principal inpatient claim	Number with no inpatient claim	Subset* with annual costs over $12K	With inpatient claim and costs > $12K		With no inpatient claim and costs > $12K	
				N	% of subset > $12K	N	% of subset > $12K
Chemotherapy	3,814	1,041	3,470	3,327	.96	143	.04
End-stage liver disorders	1,185	1,148	911	858	.94	53	.06
Asthma	26,640	200,317	7,072	5,203	.74	1,869	.26
Manic-depressive disorders	24,523	67,234	18,140	12,294	.68	5,846	.32
GI hemorrhage	2,482	17,874	2,018	1,335	.66	683	.34
Peripheral vascular disease	1,281	13,909	1,435	892	.62	543	.38
Chronic skin ulcer	1,537	11,458	1,807	1,129	.62	678	.38

Source: Data from Georgia, Tennessee, and Michigan.

* The subset with annual costs over $12,000 is selected from among those shown in the first two columns, who either had the diagnosis as a principal inpatient diagnosis or who had the diagnosis as an ambulatory diagnosis while having no inpatient claim for the year. The figures in the table thus exclude those who had the diagnosis as a non-principal inpatient diagnosis or who had the diagnosis as ambulatory but also had any hospital claim. The percentages in antepenultimate and last column show the distribution of those with and without inpatient claims among the selected subset of beneficiaries.

ulcers. Clinicians tend to agree that multiple diagnoses add substantially to complexity and cost of care.

The shift from using the single most serious diagnosis to using multiple diagnoses is one of the major differences between the first round of DCG models developed from the mid-1980s to the mid-1990s and the Hierarchical Coexisting Condition (HCC) models developed by Ash, Ellis, Pope, and colleagues (Ellis et al. 1996). Jonathan Weiner, Barbara Starfield, and colleagues (1991), who have developed the ambulatory care group (ACG) models for Medicare payments, have also used multiple diagnoses from both inpatient and ambulatory settings, as has our work on the Disability Payment System (DPS), developed for payments for Medicaid beneficiaries (Kronick and Dreyfus 1997).

Improvements in accuracy from counting multiple diagnoses can be seen in the difference between the predictive ratios for the two approaches. For example, the ADDCG model counts diagnoses made by physicians in inpatient and ambulatory settings but only the single most serious one, as in the PIPDCG model, in which one of 12 different cost levels can be assigned. The HCC model also uses diagnoses made by physicians in any setting but can use multiple diagnoses to predict future expenditures. The prospective HCC model has 34 diagnostic categories (e.g., liver disease, coronary artery disease, higher-cost pneumonia). Counting rules prevent the double counting of diagnoses that are highly related, such as congestive heart failure and coronary artery disease. As expected, the predictive ratios for validation groups that are made up of beneficiaries with a single diagnosis defined independently from the diagnostic categories are better for HCC than for ADDCG. Table 3.1 shows, for example, that for individuals with hip fractures in 1991 the ADDCG model predicts 85 percent of costs in 1992, while the HCC model predicts 99 percent of costs; for individuals with depression, ADDCG predicts 80 percent of costs, HCC 87 percent.

The use of multiple diagnoses is also supported by our finding among Medicaid beneficiaries with disability that expenditures are substantially higher for people with greater numbers of diagnoses in the previous year. Counting diagnoses in the disability payment system, we found that Medicaid beneficiaries with disability who had had only a single chronic diagnosis in 1993 had average monthly expenditures in 1994 of $370, while those with two chronic diagnoses in 1993 had average monthly expenditures in 1994 of $500. Those with five chronic diagnoses had next year average monthly costs of $990 (see Figure 3.1).

Another reason to move to collection of diagnostic data from all encounters is to support quality monitoring. The completeness of encounter-level data is increasingly needed not only for adjusting payments but

Figure 3.1 1994 Monthly Expenditures by Number of 1993 DPS Diagnoses

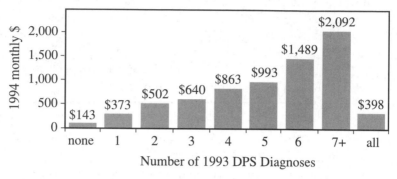

Source: Kronick, R., and T. Dreyfus. 1997. *The Challenge of Risk Adjustment for People with Disabilities: Health-Based Payment for Medicaid Programs; a Guide for State Medicaid Programs, Providers, and Consumers.* Princeton, NJ: Center for Health Care Strategies, 25.

also for monitoring quality. Making appropriate payments and monitoring quality are two sides of the larger challenge payors face in buying the greatest value for their healthcare dollars. Health-based payment using all diagnostic data will allow Medicare to identify more precisely those beneficiaries with chronic conditions or disability and to use the encounter-level data to make meaningful comparisons of utilization across plans for people with similar conditions. If payment is based only on inpatient diagnoses, then related diagnostically adjusted examinations of quality would be limited to the roughly 20 percent of beneficiaries who experience a hospitalization in a given year.

In sum, the movement to using all diagnoses is critical to making health-based payment work right. The use of all diagnoses will fix the serious incentive to hospitalize created by the use of inpatient data only. It will also make the payments substantially more accurate. Finally, the use of all diagnoses will greatly enhance the use of diagnostic information for quality monitoring purposes.

Because most diagnoses are made more frequently outside the hospital than inside, the shift to using all diagnoses brings large changes in the cost implications of most diagnoses. When the payment system switches to the use of all diagnoses, a much larger stream of diagnoses will be used to determine payments, but each diagnosis will have a smaller effect on future payments. For example, comparing diagnoses that appear in both the PIPDCG model and the ADDCG model, we see that many more people are classified as having particular diagnoses, but that the average subsequent-year costs of those with the diagnoses are lower (see Table 3.4).

Table 3.4   Average Subsequent-Year Costs for Beneficiaries
with Diagnoses Made as Principal Inpatient Diagnosis (PIPDCG)
and as Any Physician Diagnosis (ADDCG)

	Principal Inpatient		Any Physician	
Diagnosis in 1991	N	Mean $ in 1992	N	Mean $ in 1992
Heart failure	7,043	$13,096	42,021	$7,118
Ventricular tachycardia	371	10,257	3,199	8,037
Regional enteritis	178	9,201	475	3,684

Source: Ellis, R. P., et al. 1996. *Diagnostic Cost Group (DCG) and Hierarchical Coexisting Conditions (HCC) Models for Medicare Risk Adjustment, Final Report to HCFA,* Contract no. 500-92-0020, April 1996. Waltham, MA: Health Economics Research, Tables C-1 and C-2.

The Challenge of Increased Coding Frequency

A major but so far little appreciated difficulty about the use of diagnostic data is the great potential for variation in the frequency of diagnoses made and recorded for beneficiaries under different circumstances. According to preliminary analyses we and others have done, fee-for-service data shows significant under-reporting of diagnoses. Health plans being paid diagnostically adjusted rates, on the other hand, will have strong incentives to report diagnoses much more completely. Their abilities to do so, however, will vary from plan to plan.

As a result, in implementing health-based payment, Medicare may need to account for both the more complete coding by plans relative to fee-for-service and the variation in coding completeness among plans. Medicare uses its fee-for-service beneficiaries as a baseline for setting rates, so that plan members may appear sicker than the fee-for-service average only because the fee-for-service data significantly under-report diagnoses.[7]

Work with Medicaid data shows that chronic diagnoses that appear in an individual's claims in one 12-month period often do not appear in the subsequent 12-month period. For example, among SSI beneficiaries with a diagnosis of quadriplegia in their fee-for-service claims during a given year, only 55 percent have a diagnosis of quadriplegia appear in claims in the following year. While some diagnoses show a fairly high level of year-to-year persistence (e.g., schizophrenia at 84 percent) many chronic diagnoses persist at approximately the 60 percent level, and some are even lower.[8] As may be expected, among beneficiaries who have a given diagnosis in the first year, those whose diagnoses persist have much higher second-year costs than those whose diagnoses do not persist. The Medicare Payment Advisory Committee found very similar results: among Medicare beneficiaries with a variety of chronic diagnoses in fee-for-service claims in 1994, only

50 to 60 percent also had the same chronic diagnosis in 1995 (MedPAC 1998b, 16–17).

What a "correct" level of persistence would be for various diagnoses cannot be empirically determined from claims. But it seems very likely that a much higher degree of persistence would be seen for chronic conditions if plan clinicians were encouraged to code more fully. HCFA guidelines for the use of International Classification of Disease codes suggest "Chronic disease(s) treated on an ongoing basis may be coded and reported as many times as the patient receives treatment and care for the condition" (ICD 1997, 14–16). In addition to the condition that is the reason for the encounter, clinicians should "Code all documented conditions that coexist at the time of the visit that require or affect patient care, treatment or management." A physician seeing a beneficiary with paraplegia because of a skin ulcer, urinary tract infection or a mental health problem could quite appropriately indicate paraplegia as a coexisting condition. Most serious chronic illnesses and disabilities can reasonably be identified for many healthcare encounters as a coexisting condition that affects "care, treatment or management." When plans are paid on the basis of diagnoses, we would expect that many more beneficiaries would be diagnosed with chronic conditions.

Plans could not reasonably report that all diagnoses recorded in the previous year persist into the current year. The guidelines offer a fairly straightforward limit: "Do not code conditions that were previously treated and no longer exist." But plans could reasonably move from the 60 to 80 percent persistence we see in fee-for-service claims up toward a full report of chronic diagnoses with persistence perhaps in the range of 75 to 100 percent, depending on the condition. Much of the improvement in reporting could come from a relatively simple software system that would remind physicians at each visit of all the diagnoses that had been made for the member in the previous year. Physicians could then simply check off those conditions that still coexisted with the reason for the visit. While auditing of diagnostic reports by clinicians working for Medicare is needed to limit fraudulent coding, we anticipate that most of the change in coding will be perfectly legitimate and demands a careful response in order to maintain budget neutrality and fairness of payments among plans. If payment amounts were developed on fee-for-service data but plans report diagnoses more frequently, then the payment amounts based directly on plan diagnoses and fee-for-service weights would lead to overpayments.

Adjusting for Changes in Diagnostic Reporting

HCFA can solve this problem by measuring and adjusting for changes in diagnostic reporting. If plans are evaluating their members as 10 percent sicker than these same members were in fee-for-service arrangements, then payment rates need to be adjusted downward to get the payment right. Because large numbers of beneficiaries continue to move from fee-for-service into health plans, it would not be difficult to compare the case-mix of beneficiaries before and after the switch. The proportion of this change that results from increased diagnostic reporting needs to be removed from the case mix estimates for each plan.

Most, but not all, of the increased case mix will result from increased intensity of diagnostic reporting. A small amount of this change, however, will result from beneficiaries actually getting sicker over time, and this needs to be netted out of the overall change. This real change in health status can easily be estimated by comparing the case mix of a large group of beneficiaries in fee-for-service in one year with the case mix of the same individuals who are still in fee-for-service the next year. One could also look at plan members from year to year. Medicare can calculate these real changes, perhaps separately for different age groups, and subtract them from the overall estimate of case-mix change.

One potential problem is that plans may differ substantially in how quickly they can move to full reporting. If some plans were particularly slow in getting their clinicians to report diagnoses, then they would get unfairly lower payments with an industry-wide adjustment for increased reporting. Yet calculating reporting adjustments separately for each plan would be difficult and would reward plans for their failure to report fully.

Alternatively, the use of ambulatory data could be phased in over several years, with an industry-wide adjustment for increased diagnostic reporting. This approach would keep the pressure on plans to make full diagnostic reports but would give them more time to learn how to do so, with modest financial losses for failing to do so in the first year growing over the phase-in period. For example, the first year in which ambulatory diagnoses are used, the payment could be based 75 percent on principal inpatient diagnosis only, 25 percent on all diagnoses, with a 25 percent increase on the weight of all diagnoses in the next three years.

The Challenge to Plans

Implementation of health-based payment will depend on the ability of health plans to report their members' diagnoses, and some health plans are understandably concerned that health-based payment will require substantial new investment in information systems. Many plans can adapt their information systems to report diagnoses with a fairly modest effort, while others will need to make large improvements. Yet a buyer of managed care services should not hesitate to insist that plans know and report the most basic health information that is required in any case for quality improvement—the chronic diagnoses of the members whose care they are supposed to be managing.

Although the Balanced Budget Act has given HCFA substantial authority to move ahead, resistance from health plans may still greatly slow the process or dilute the final product. Health plans are understandably concerned about health-based payment, because it will reduce payments to some plans, increase payments to those that attract people with greater needs, while requiring all to make reports of Medicare members' diagnoses. But the reorientation of the healthcare industry toward a more systematic focus on quality is a goal that all participants can embrace. Such an important change cannot come without difficulty, but the results should amply reward the effort.

OPTIONS FOR DIAGNOSTIC ADJUSTMENT

Alternative Classification Systems

While initial implementation of health-based payment will use the PIPDCG model, HCFA still must decide what classification system to use for ongoing implementation. The system used for ongoing health-based payment will most likely be one that uses diagnoses and perhaps other information from care provided in the hospital and at ambulatory sites.

HCFA has invested substantial support for the two types of models that use multiple diagnoses: the Ambulatory Care Group models developed by Weiner, Starfield, and colleagues (1991), and the Hierarchical Coexisting Condition models developed by Ash, Ellis, Pope, and colleagues (Ellis et al. 1996), who had previously developed the DCG models. Other models are also available, including the Disability Payment System, which we developed for Medicaid programs, but which also appears, in preliminary analysis, to work very well for Medicare beneficiaries.

The *Ambulatory Care Group (ACG) approach* was originally developed to predict ambulatory care needs among a general population (Weiner et al. 1991), but has more recently incorporated inpatient diagnoses to help predict total expenditures among Medicare beneficiaries. One virtue of the ACG approach is that its broader categories capture many Medicare beneficiaries—for example, "major signs and symptoms" (31 percent of beneficiaries) and "discrete likely to recur" (24 percent)—so that the system does well in distinguishing people who are sick in any way from those who have no conditions needing care (Weiner et al. 1996).

On the other hand, many diagnoses that appear in other systems to have quite different effects on future expenditures are assigned to the same ambulatory diagnostic category. As a result, most of the categories are predictive for Medicare beneficiaries of only small amounts of additional expenditures: most of the ambulatory categories have annual weights of under

$1,000, and even most of the hospital-based major diagnostic categories have effects only in the range of $1,000 to $4,000. These modest coefficients when the ACG system is estimated on the Medicare population limit the accuracy of prediction, especially for higher-cost individuals, whose degree of need is not distinguished from those with a moderate level of need. The developers of the ACG system, however, have worked actively to revise their model, devoting more detailed attention, for example, to predicting costs for beneficiaries with multiple diagnoses (Johns Hopkins 1998).

The *Hierarchical Coexisting Conditions (HCG) model* uses a large number of diagnostic groups, some of which are narrowly defined to help better fit the conditions of the over-65 population. Among the 34 diagnostic categories are groups as specific as bone infections, respiratory failure, congestive heart failure, and coma. A number of conditions are divided into categories by degree of severity—for example, cancers, gastrointestinal conditions, pneumonias, and diabetes are each divided into two or three categories according to cost level. Individuals with diagnoses in more than one level of the same kind of condition are assigned only to the more costly category.

Compared with the generally broader categories of the ACG models, the finer HCC categories select narrower groups of people with predictably higher costs. In fitting the model to a large sample of Medicare beneficiaries, nine of the HCC categories had coefficients near or over $4,000.

The *Disability Payment System* (DPS) was developed to allow states to adjust payments to health plans that enroll Medicaid beneficiaries with disability or chronic illness. DPS is fairly similar to the HCC model in general design. Diagnoses associated with elevated future costs are divided into 18 major categories, most of which are further divided according to the degree of elevated future costs, which produces 43 subcategories. DPS always counts multiple diagnoses from different major categories, but not always within major categories. In some major categories only the most serious diagnosis is counted, while in others counting of multiple diagnoses is allowed. Like the HCC categories and unlike the ACG categories, a number of the DPS subcategories identify quite tightly defined groups of individuals with costs substantially above average.

Chris Hogan of the Medicare Payment Advisory Commission staff has done preliminary work with DPS using 1994 diagnoses of Medicare beneficiaries to predict their 1995 costs. He found R^2 statistics of .16 for beneficiaries under age 65 and .11 for those aged 65 or over. While a variety of differences in methods make these analyses not directly comparable to those of the HCC models, Ellis and Ash report R^2 statistics of .12 for under-65 beneficiaries and .08 for beneficiaries age 65 or over (Ellis et al. 1996a,

Table F-4). More work is needed to understand the differences between the performance of the two models, but it is intriguing that DPS performed as well as the HCC model for older beneficiaries and far better for beneficiaries with disability.

Prospective versus Concurrent Adjustment

Research in health-based payment has focused most on predicting future resource needs, with payment weights based on the association between diagnoses in one year and expenditures in the next year. Yet there are potential advantages to using *concurrent* weights, which are calculated by regressing expenditures for one year against diagnoses made in the same year. At least on an individual basis, concurrent assessment varies payment to match needs more accurately, with much higher R^2 statistics. Significant questions remain, however, about concurrent adjustment in terms of both the selection of diagnoses and the timing of assessment and payment. Done wrong, concurrent adjustment could offer incentives to hospitalize that appear far too strong; done right, it may offer more accurate payments and a positive compromise between the incentives of fee-for-service and capitation.

The estimated costs associated concurrently with many diagnoses are much higher than diagnoses in prospective regressions. (These higher weights for diagnoses draw money away from the baseline or the age-gender payments so that the total payments estimated for the population are the same.) The effects on payment weights from switching to a concurrent framework are most dramatic when looking only at principal inpatient diagnoses. In the case of the PIPDCG model, the number of diagnoses that are associated with costs over $20,000 jumps from two in the prospective version (chemotherapy at $23,700 and end-stage liver disorders at $20,900) to 41 in the concurrent model, including 14 over $30,000 (Ellis et al. 1996b, Tables C-1 and C-5). Thus, adjusting payments on a concurrent basis using only principal inpatient diagnoses would seem to offer extremely large and inappropriate incentives to hospitalize. We believe that concurrent adjustment should not be used when adjustment is by inpatient diagnoses only and is considered an option only when inpatient and ambulatory diagnoses are used for adjustment.

The much higher R^2 statistics that are seen for concurrent models must be regarded with caution. These statistics suggest that concurrent models track individual expenditures much more closely than predictive models, but much of the improvement is simply a result of the powerful association between current diagnoses and current expenditures, even when random and unpredictable. Concurrent regressions are only predicting what has already happened, in effect describing the increased current costs of people with expensive diagnoses. These higher R^2 statistics of concurrent models do not translate into systematically better predictions in year two for biased groups defined in year one.[9]

CHANGES IN THE BALANCED BUDGET ACT, INCLUDING OLD AND NEW APPROACHES TO GEOGRAPHY

Changes in Setting Capitation Rates

In addition to starting down the path of health-based payment, the Balanced Budget Act brings a host of other important changes to the setting of Medicare capitation rates. Notably, the act mandates changes in how geographical variation and growth of healthcare expenditures are incorporated into capitation rates. Although these issues are fairly distinct from health-based payment, all the new methods will also interact to produce the final rates.

These changes can be seen as part of a package of changes intended to correct longstanding defects in Medicare payment methods. The changes include:

- *A blend of national and local rates.* Local rates will be progressively blended with a national rate, which will tend to compress extreme rates toward the national average. In 1998, the blend will be 90 percent local and 10 percent national. The national proportion of the blend will increase 8 percent each year, until it reaches 50 percent in 2003. Because of minimum rates and minimum increases, however, the blended rates will only begin to be used in 2000, likely spreading to most counties over the period 2001–2003 (MedPAC 1998a).

- *Price adjustment of the national rate.* For the blending, a single national capitation rate will first be set at the average of the local rates. This national rate will then be adjusted for local input prices to create a price-adjusted national rate in each county that will be blended with the local rate.

- *Local rates based on 1997 rates updated for spending growth.* The 1997 AAPCC rates will be used as the basis for the future local rates, which will no longer depend on future local fee-for-service expenditures. The act sets future growth for the local rates at national Medicare spending growth, but for 1998 sets growth at 0.8 percent less and for 1999–2002 sets growth at 0.5 percent less than national Medicare growth.[10]

- *Alternative minimum rates and minimum increases.* The act also creates a minimum rate, $367 in 1998, that will be paid instead of a lower national-local blend. This floor will rise each year with the same percentage growth as is used for the local rates. In addition, the 1997 rate in each area will be inflated 2 percent each year to calculate a minimum increase and will be paid if it is higher than the blended rate or the floor rate for the area.

These significant changes will interact with others. Expenditures to support medical training will be removed from the 1997 rates that form the basis for future rates. It was argued that health plans were not necessarily contracting with or passing on these funds to teaching hospitals. This reduction of expenditures for medical education will be made gradually, in annual decrements of one-fifth from 1998 to 2002. The blended rates will also be adjusted overall to ensure budget neutrality, that is, that the payments made under the blended rates will not exceed the payments that would have been made under the area-specific rates.

The combination of all these changes and the implementation of health-based payment should allow health plans to enroll members with a greater range of healthcare needs in a wider variety of places. But they are also designed to reduce longstanding overpayments to plans for healthier than average beneficiaries and for residents of certain metropolitan areas. These reductions in payment are likely to aggravate the concerns of plans and beneficiaries about the adequacy of Medicare capitation payments.

Over time, the number of zero-premium plans and the extent of free supplemental benefits may well be reduced. Thus, the changes in financing could bring discontent that may fall onto health-based payment if the effects of changes in how geographical variation and growth of expenditures are handled are attributed to health-based payment. The sections below examine the issues behind some of the changes.

Reducing Geographical Variation

Since 1985 HCFA has been setting different Medicare capitation rates for each county in the nation based on fee-for-service expenditures and demographic characteristics of beneficiaries in the county. The Adjusted Average Per Capita Cost (AAPCC) estimated what the fee-for-service costs would be in the county for a beneficiary with demographic risk factors at the national average. To achieve savings from managed care, the base county rates were set at 95 percent of the AAPCC. The actual payments to plans, however, were a proportion or multiple of the base county rate that depended on the age and other demographic characteristics of each plan's members.

The insufficiency of demographic information to estimate risk was discussed earlier. But the use of fee-for-service expenditures by county also created problems. The most obvious problem has been that the county rates vary too much. As a result, beneficiaries in some areas have plenty of Medicare plans to choose from, while beneficiaries in others areas have few or none. Monthly county rates in 1997 ranged from a high of $767 to a low of $221. Some of this range results from higher urban and lower rural expenditures, but even among central urban counties, rates varied from $767 to $349. Substantial rate variation is found even within single metropolitan areas that are composed of multiple counties, for example in the St. Louis area, with a range from $542 to $377 (PPRC 1997, 44–45).

In high-rate counties, plans have more than enough money to cover costs and are devoting funds toward supplemental benefits and reduction or elimination of member premiums. In low-rate counties, if plans are available, supplemental benefits are much more limited and members must pay substantial premiums. It appears to be quite unfair that in Miami beneficiaries receive drug and dental benefits and pay no premium for coverage, while in Portland, Oregon, beneficiaries rarely get these extra benefits and are paying substantial premiums (PPRC 1997, 49–50).

The blending of national and local rates should do much to reduce the problem of excessive geographic rate spread. The blending and the minimum should increase the availability and choice of health plans in low-rate areas and reduce the unfair disparity of supplemental benefits and premiums.

But it is fair to ask, how will a compressed rate system address the *causes* of the county variation? Some of the county variation resulted from risk differences that were missed by demographic factors and that diagnostic factors will better capture. Some of the county variation resulted from differences in local input prices, which will be reflected by the blending of local rates with a national rate adjusted to local prices. Some of the variation also resulted from differences in practice patterns, for which Medicare should perhaps not be paying (though Medicare is paying for it in fee-for-service, which makes appropriate HMO rate setting difficult). The compression of the county rates should reduce payments in areas where services have been provided too eagerly and increase resources where services have been underprovided.

Locking In the Relative County Rates

Another problem that the Balanced Budget Act attempts to fix is the variability of rates over time. By establishing the 1997 rates as the basis for future rates, the BBA locks in the relative levels of the 1997 rates from county to county. A ranking of the counties by rate should be quite consistent over time, because their relative positions will not be changed by the compression of the range caused by the minimum rate and the local-national blending. (The gradually increasing removal of funds for medical education will cause some shift in the ranking as the counties with larger expenditures in their rates will fall slightly in comparison with other counties.)

Locking in the relative positions of the county rates also addresses a more subtle but more important problem in the relationship between county fee-for-service expenditures and capitation rates. Formerly, HCFA used five-year moving averages of county fee-for-service expenditures, projected forward through changes in national expenditures from inflation and benefit changes. This use of county fee-for-service expenditures as the basis for county capitation rates rested on the assumption that beneficiaries in fee-for-service were equivalent to beneficiaries in managed care once adjustments were made for demographic factors.

As reviewed in Chapter 2, several studies have found, however, that HMOs have enjoyed favorable selection within the demographic risk groups. This favorable selection may or may not moderate over time as managed care becomes more established. In the many areas where managed care enrollment is growing, the fee-for-service and managed care groups may often diverge into higher and lower cost groups.

Effects of Diagnostic Adjustment on the Local Rates

A complex issue is how the use of diagnostic risk adjustment will affect the base local rates and the actual payments. It appears that the adoption of health-based payment will further compress the local base rates, though not necessarily the actual rates paid to plans, which will depend increasingly on the health status of a plan's members. A quick foray is needed into how the AAPCC's national risk categories have been used with local demographic risk data to produce actual rates paid to plans based on their enrollment. The technique of using national adjusters to create payments that reflect both local costs and plan enrollment will still be required with diagnostic-based payment.

The past county AAPCCs were not simply the projected fee-for-service expenditures for actual beneficiaries in the county but the projected expenditures in the county for an individual with the *national* average level of risk. The "Adjusted" of the Adjusted Average Per Capita Cost refers to the adjustment needed to estimate the costs in the county of the national average risk beneficiary. By calculating a rate in each county for the national average risk beneficiary, HCFA could then use risk factors based on large national populations. The national demographic factors were used to calculate the risk of a plan's enrollees relative to the national average. The assessed level of risk for the plan could then be multiplied by the projected costs for a national average risk in the county to reach a fair payment.

Algebra may clarify. The first fraction in the formula below represents the adjustment to get from actual projected per capita (p.c.) county expenditures to the AAPCC, or the average expenditures in the county for a national average risk, and the second fraction represents the final step to get the plan payment:

$$\text{payment} = \text{projected p.c. county spending} \times .95 \times \frac{\text{national risk}}{\text{county risk}} \times \frac{\text{plan risk}}{\text{national risk}}$$

Simplifying, we see that the final payment is:

$$\text{payment} = \text{projected p.c. county spending} \times .95 \times \frac{\text{plan risk}}{\text{county risk}}$$

In other words, through the national risk factors, the final payment to a plan is the projected per capita spending in the county, boosted or diminished according to the degree by which the plan's risk is greater or less than the county risk. This is just the right result.

The result of this method of calculation is that the per capita costs in a county with a disproportionate share of older beneficiaries would be reduced to get an AAPCC that would represent the costs in that county of serving the national average risk beneficiary. But the payment to a plan would depend on its enrollment. If a plan enrolled membership that was representative of the county age mix and older than the national average beneficiary, it would get paid more than the county AAPCC.

The same logic needs to be followed in the implementation of health-based payment. Like the traditional demographic risk factors, the diagnostic risk assessment is based on national relationships between diagnoses and expenditures. The projected per capita county spending levels are being replaced by 1997 county spending levels, trended upward and gradually compressed by the minimum and the national-local blending. But the resulting spending levels in each county will need to be adjusted by the diagnostic risk in each county in order to use national diagnosis-based risk factors to set plan rates.

Because demographic risk differences appear to account for only a modest amount of variation in expenditures, the demographic adjustment of county expenditures had only a modest effect in reducing the actual average expenditures from counties with above-average risk to a slightly lower AAPCC. For example, Dade County's 1995 average Medicare per capita cost of $687 was only moderately reduced by a demographic risk index of 1.06 to an AAPCC of $648 and a rate of $616 (95 percent of $648). At the low end of the range, Hennepin County's $378 in actual spending was hardly changed by a demographic risk index of .99 to an AAPCC of $382 and a rate of $363 (PPRC 1997, 57).[11]

With much more effective diagnostic risk adjustment, however, we can expect a much more substantial compression of the local rates. Using the HCC model, for example, to create a diagnosis-based index comparable to the demographic index leads to a significant narrowing of rate variation. Dade's diagnostic index was a high 1.34, which would reduce the $616 base rate to a $459 diagnosis-adjusted base rate. By contrast, Hennepin County's .89 diagnostic index boosted its $363 base rate to $408 (PPRC 1997, 63).[12] The diagnostic adjustment lowers Dade's apparent 1.7 times higher cost relative to Hennepin down to only 1.13 times higher. The HCC indexes for the metropolitan areas of Los Angeles (1.13), Detroit (1.23), New York (1.05), and Philadelphia (1.15) suggest that these areas would see substantial base rate reduction, while Milwaukee (.95), Seattle (.91), and a number of rural areas such as in Wisconsin (.90) would have substantial base rate increases.

Although diagnostic risk adjustment will substantially squeeze base rates, it will not necessarily squeeze the final payments—those will depend greatly on enrollment. The data above suggest that much of the higher expenditures and higher demographic-based base rates are due to real differences in health risk. The base rates, however, reflect the costs of care for the *national* average health risk beneficiary. If a plan in Miami enrolls beneficiaries who as a group have the same level of high health risk as Dade County as a whole, it will get paid substantially more than the Dade base rate.

On the other hand, if the plan enrolls a healthier group, say a group with a health risk like the national average, it will get paid the more modest Dade average now adjusted to reflect the national average healthcare risk if served in Dade County. This is just what health-based payment is supposed to do, but it means real reductions for plans that have been enjoying undeserved profits of favorable selection.

The Balanced Budget Act does not specify how the risk adjustment would interact with the blending and the minimum increases. This ambiguity creates a potential for health plans to argue that the final county base rates should not be lower than the budget-neutral blends of local and national rates; that is, that diagnostic risk adjustment should not lead to any loss of revenues regardless of their enrollees' risk status. But the area-specific portion of the blend and probably also the rates based on the minimum have to be divided by the county average risk to reach a county average adjusted to reflect the national average risk.[13] Only in this way can the nationally developed risk adjusters and the risk scores of each plan's enrollment be applied to calculate the risk-appropriate payment for the plan.

Implications for the Role of Managed Care

The extent to which diagnostic adjustment reins in the extremes of the rates presents something of a challenge to current thinking in health economics. The strong reduction of expenditure variation by diagnostic adjustment means that diagnoses appear to account for much of the differences among areas in health expenditures. The average 75-year-old man in Miami may in fact be substantially sicker than the 75-year-old man in Minneapolis.

If this finding holds, it would appear to contradict an important prevailing view among health economists who have supported managed care. The small-area studies of Wennberg and others concluded that substantial variation in practice patterns among different areas is not justified by differences in burden of illness (Wennberg 1998; Fisher et al. 1994). Practice pattern variation has instead been attributed to inappropriate variation in physician judgment or resource availability—variation that should be reduced for a more efficient healthcare system. This prevailing understanding has supported the view that managed care organizations have a valuable role to play in their potential to detect and reduce unjustified variation in practice patterns. Were earlier studies perhaps relying on measures of illness burden that were too crude? Are detailed diagnostic profiles shedding new light? To what degree are the diagnoses themselves dependent on variation in physician judgment and in resource availability?

ADJUSTING FOR PROVISION OF END-OF-LIFE CARE

Even with diagnostic adjustment of payments, a good case could be made for the addition of mortality rates as a basis for adjustment. As noted above, the 5 percent of Medicare beneficiaries who die each year account for approximately 30 percent of Medicare expenditures. Prospective adjustment by diagnoses will tend to predict only a small portion of these expenditures, because very few diagnoses made in one year prove fatal to a significant proportion of individuals in the following year.

A plan that does a particularly good job at end-of-life care and attracts a disproportionate share of Medicare beneficiaries close to the end of their lives would almost certainly not be compensated adequately by a system that adjusted payment only by diagnosis and demographic factors. Conversely, a plan that attracts disproportionately few beneficiaries needing end-of-life care would earn undeserved profits. In addition to more equitably compensating plans for their members' healthcare needs, paying for end-of-life care that meets certain standards could lead to much-needed improvements in its quality.

Given current enrollment patterns and mortality rates, simply adjusting for mortality would substantially reduce payments to the average plan with low mortality, perhaps by about 5 percent. As reviewed in Chapter 2, a variety of studies have shown that mortality rates in HMOs are approximately 80 percent of mortality rates in fee-for-service. The combination of the high costs of end-of-life care and the lower mortality rate in plans creates a 5 percent difference in expected costs. Further, mortality rates among new HMO enrollees are lower than mortality rates among longer-term enrollees. As a result, where managed care enrollment is increasing, the disparity in mortality rates is also growing.

We believe that serious attention has not been paid to the possibility of adjusting payment for mortality because it would appear to be "paying for death," which would provide an incentive for plans to let members die. We think, however, that mortality adjustment could play a very positive role in providing incentives to improve end-of-life care if it were coupled with strong measures to improve quality. We propose:

1. that plans be paid using diagnostic-based payment with large additional payments for beneficiaries who die; and
2. that these additional payments be made *only* to plans that are certified by HCFA as meeting high standards for end-of-life care.

The details of such standards would need to be developed carefully, but we imagine that they would include protocols for discussion of end-of-life care among caregivers, beneficiaries, and their families; provisions for hospice care; and training of providers in pain management and terminal care. To be certified, plans would need to have a sample of deaths reviewed annually to see that care had actually met the standards. Because plans would have great difficulty surviving financially if they received none of the payments for end-of-life care, a graduated scale of penalties should be imposed on plans that only partially meet the standards.

Concerns about "paying for death" parallel the objection that diagnostic adjustment will discourage plans from treating or preventing illness. The common element is a concern that payment for negative events such as illness or death will discourage plans from taking steps to prevent illness and death. But these concerns appear misplaced, because the vast majority of medical care is about responding to illness, including extreme illness that leads to death. Clinicians have only limited influence on whether people get sick or when they die, and plan decisions have even less effect. A plan with a disproportionate mortality rate or a disproportionate share of members who are sick is likely not doing something wrong—it is more likely to be doing something right in order to attract and retain members with such greater needs, and it should be paid accordingly.

Imagine the case of an individual who has been struggling for some years with a worsening heart condition or with cancer and who is now deteriorating dangerously. The therapeutic approach pursued by the individual's caregivers may make the difference between the person dying within months or living for another year. The choice of approach should result from decision making by the individual and family members who have been informed by clinicians about the likely outcomes of different approaches. Despite recent efforts to promote patient and family understanding and participation in the choices presented by end-of-life care, the current state of medicine unfortunately is far from this ideal (Schneiderman and Jecker 1995). (We note also the current unfortunate regulations that require beneficiaries to disenroll from plans in order to receive hospice services.)

Payment thus presents one way the Medicare program could strongly support the movement toward more informed patient involvement in decisions about end-of-life care. Medicare could make a substantial payment to cover end-of-life care for each enrolled beneficiary who dies, provided that the plan can meet standards of quality for end-of-life care, such as appropriate involvement of clinicians with the beneficiary in discussion of care options. Payments for end-of-life care could also be varied according to the cause of death, so that a plan with a member who died a sudden death may receive little additional payment while a plan that provided extensive care for someone dying of cancer, Alzheimer's, or heart disease may be paid substantially.

It is hard to see that a payment for providing end-of-life care would cause plans to let their members die too easily, because the payment will come sooner or later. Of course, in any system of capitated payments, plans face incentives to under-provide, and these concerns are naturally heightened for terminal care. Individuals are extremely vulnerable as they approach the end of life and often have little capacity for self-advocacy or decision making. But the observation about incentives to under-provide supports the argument that full-risk capitation be softened through risk sharing or partial capitation so as to make the plan indifferent to additional spending; it is not an argument against paying for end-of-life care. Far from creating incentives to let people die quickly, payments for end-of-life care only in plans that provide it with high quality should reduce the incentives to under-provide.

The concern about "paying for death" is reasonable in some circumstances. Some individuals are gravely ill but recover after very costly treatments and live many additional years. Some such individuals may be so critically ill that they appear to be dying. Although it would be extremely contrary to medical ethics, a plan could be tempted by a payment for mortality to skip the costly measures and let the member die. The plan would save the large expenses and could receive a large payment for end-of-life care, depending on the cause of death and assuming the plan was certified in end-of-life care. Thus careful monitoring would be needed, including detailed sample reviews of cases, in order to prevent this kind of abuse. Plans that lost certification as responsible providers of end-of-life care would face large financial losses and may well be unable to continue serving Medicare beneficiaries.

Policymakers have not focused much discussion or research on the possibility of paying more for end-of-life care, no doubt concerned about the possibility of headlines such as "Feds Pay HMOs to Kill Elders." But the positive side of this approach may become more evident as more attention is paid in general to service quality and specifically to the importance of care that is sensitive to the needs and wishes of people who are dying. Adjustment by mortality also makes sense because it is far simpler to do than adjustment by diagnoses, which are often not clear-cut.

If political problems prevent adjustment by mortality rates, they would still prove a very valuable confirmation of the appropriateness of rates adjusted only by diagnoses. Plans that have a disproportionately high share of chronic illness will likely have a high mortality rate, just as plans with a disproportionately low share of chronic illness should have low mortality rates. To the extent that mortality rates confirm the results of diagnostic assessment, it will be difficult for plans to argue that apparent variations in risk across plans are largely caused by variations in coding instead of by real variation in illness.

SUMMARY

Implementation of an effective system of health-based payment is a critical step in orienting the healthcare industry toward providing high-quality care for the chronically ill and solving the problems raised by risk selection. The BBA provides HCFA with a legislative mandate to move forward, and HCFA is working diligently to implement this mandate. As of the spring of 1998, however, even limited implementation of health-based payment using only inpatient hospital data in 2000 is far from certain. Some HMOs are resisting providing the necessary data; the BBA language "freezing" the 1997 rate book may make it difficult for HCFA to implement health-based payment in a manner that effectively deals with geographic variation in the AAPCC; and HCFA is still scrambling to secure the administrative resources necessary to process the stream of hospital discharge data that the BBA requires HMOs to provide.

Assuming that HCFA can solve these immediate problems, it is important that it move quickly to expand the assessment of health status to the use of both inpatient and ambulatory diagnoses, as has been done recently by a number of state Medicaid programs. Relying solely on inpatient diagnoses penalizes those plans that have worked aggressively to move care out of the hospital into the community and creates incentives for plans to reengineer healthcare delivery to focus more on inpatient care. Relying only on inpatient data provides little assurance, in the long run, that plans with sicker members will be paid appropriately. Adding diagnostic information from ambulatory care to the assessment of health status will increase the reporting burden on plans, the administrative burden on HCFA, and the need to measure and adjust for accuracy in diagnostic reporting. However, the benefits from fostering the development of high-quality, efficient systems of care and rewarding the plans that attract those most in need should far outweigh the costs.

Paying plans for high-quality end-of-life care offers a simple method of health-based payment that HCFA should consider as a supplement to the use of diagnostic information in health status assessment. Policymakers may be concerned that adjusting payments to plans based on the number of beneficiaries who die may appear to be "paying for death," creating the wrong incentives and negative publicity. However, if HCFA develops a system for measuring the quality of care provided to those who die (including demonstration of improved communication among caregivers, patients, and families) and pays plans only for high-quality end-of-life care, such a system could be expected to lead to substantial improvements in care for the terminally ill.

Health-based payment is necessary, but not sufficient, to foster the development of high-quality systems of care. No capitated payment system can adjust payments so precisely that the payments for each beneficiary will reflect the expected healthcare needs of that individual. Within any "rate cell" there will always be some beneficiaries who need more care than average, and others who need less care than average. If health plans have available to them a variety of strategies—such as selective marketing, the tailoring of benefit packages, creating roadblocks or hassles for those most in need, and producing poor outcomes or otherwise subtly encouraging disenrollment of the chronically ill—they are likely to be able to achieve a favorable selection of risks, placing both taxpayers and chronically ill beneficiaries in jeopardy. The remaining chapters in this book describe and assess the effects of complementary strategies that HCFA may employ to improve care provided by plans to the chronically ill and those most in need and to limit the ability of plans to select favorable risks.

NOTES

1. Calculated from 1997 risk adjustment factors for non-Medicaid non-institutionalized beneficiaries Parts A and B with current Part A average of $298 and Part B of $169.

2. Ellis 1996b, Table F4, HCC model for aged subsample estimates for 65- to 69-year-old man with liver disease $5,577 (annual 1992 dollars), or 3.6 times the payment for same age man with no chronic condition of $1,555. Both figures include intercept of $1,192 and age-sex adjustment of $363. With liver disease and congestive heart failure, the total estimate would be $8,643, or more than 5.5 times the base.

3. The Balanced Budget Act appears to allow such experimentation without additional legislative changes. The act appears generally to favor full-risk arrangements, mandating "full financial risk" for Medicare plans and additional prospective payment systems for rehab hospitals, nursing homes, and home health agencies. At the same time, however, the act allows that Medicare plans may get reinsurance for costs beyond some level to be specified by the Secretary of Health and Human Services or for up to 90 percent of costs beyond 115 percent of its annual income.

4. See Ellis (1996b) Table 4-3 for costs and Table C-1 for frequency of beneficiaries in the categories.

5. HCFA (1998) gives 1992 Parts A and B combined USPCC of $320 and 1999 estimate of $475, for a 48 percent increase.

6. The figures thus exclude beneficiaries who had the diagnoses only as a non-principal inpatient diagnosis or who had them as an ambulatory diagnosis while having any inpatient claim for the year.

7. Medicare Payment Advisory Commission (1998a, 32) discusses this issue at some length.

8. Our analysis of Medicaid claims from Georgia, Michigan, and Tennessee.

9. See predictive ratios for concurrent models in Kronick (1996, 21) or Ellis (1996a, 115).

10. The 0.8 percent and 0.5 percent reductions helped achieve budgetary constraint that was part of the overall goal of the Balanced Budget Act. It would not be surprising if Congress decided to continue these reductions further into the future.

11. Data not identical to actual rates because of different methods of calculation.

12. The diagnosis-based index was calculated for metropolitan areas.

13. MedPAC (1998b, 23) suggests that the local part of the blend needs adjustment, but not the national. "Risk adjustment relative to the fee-for-service baseline would apply to the portion of payment that remains based on local fee-for-service costs." Their footnote suggests that the treatment of national costs, local 1997 costs, and floor payment should be specified separately.

REFERENCES

Ellis R. P., G. C. Pope, L. I. Iezzoni, J. Z. Ayanian, D. W. Bates, H. Burstin, and A. S. Ash. 1996a. "Diagnosis-Based Risk Adjustment for Medicare Capitation Payments." *Health Care Financing Review* 17 (3): 101–28.

Ellis R. P., G. C. Pope, L. I. Iezzoni, J. Z. Ayanian, D. W. Bates, H. Burstin, D. A. Dayhoff, A. Rensko, T. Dawes and A. S. Ash. 1996b. *Diagnostic Cost Group (DCG) and Hier-*

archical Coexisting Conditions (HCC) Models for Medicare Risk Adjustment, Final Report. Waltham, MA: Health Economics Research.

Enthoven, A. C. 1988. *Theory and Practice of Managed Competition in Health Care Finance.* New York: North Holland.

Fisher, E., J. Wennberg, T. Stukel, and S. Sharp. 1994. "Hospital Readmission Rates for Cohorts of Medicare Beneficiaries in Boston and New Haven." *New England Journal of Medicine* 331 (15): 989–95.

Gruenberg, L., E. Kaganova, and M. C. Hornbrook. 1996. "Improving the AAPCC with Health-Status Measures from the MCBS." *Health Care Financing Review* 17 (3): 59–76.

Health Care Financing Administration. 1998. Memo to Medicare contractors, March 2.

International Classification of Diseases, 9th Revision, Clinical Modification, Fifth Edition, 1998. 1997. Los Angeles: Practice Management Information Corp.

Johns Hopkins University ACG Case Mix Adjustment System, Documentation for PC-DOS and Unix, Version 4.1. 1998. Baltimore: Johns Hopkins University.

Kronick, R., T. Dreyfus, L. Lee, and Z. Zhou. 1996. "Diagnostic Risk Adjustment for Medicaid: The Disability Payment System." *Health Care Financing Review* 17 (3): 7–34.

Kronick, R., and T. Dreyfus. 1997. *The Challenge of Risk Adjustment for People with Disabilities: Health-Based Payment for Medicaid Programs; a Guide for State Medicaid Programs, Providers, and Consumers.* Princeton, NJ: Center for Health Care Strategies.

Lubitz, J., and G. F. Riley. 1993. "Trends in Medicare Payments in the Last Year of Life." *The New England Journal of Medicine* 328 (15): 1092–96.

Medicare Payment Advisory Commission (MedPAC). 1998a. *Report to the Congress: Medicare Payment Policy, Volume I: Recommendations.* Washington, DC.

Medicare Payment Advisory Commission (MedPAC). 1998b. *Report to the Congress: Medicare Payment Policy, Volume II: Analytical Papers.* Washington, DC.

Newhouse, J. A., M. B. Buntin, and J. D. Chapman. 1997. "Risk Adjustment and Medicare: Taking a Closer Look." *Health Affairs* 16 (5): 26–43.

Pauly, M. 1980. *Doctors and Their Workshops.* Chicago: University of Chicago Press.

Physician Payment Review Commission (PPRC). 1996. *Annual Report to Congress.* Washington, DC.

Physician Payment Review Commission (PPRC). 1997. *Annual Report to Congress.* Washington, DC.

Schneiderman, L. J., and N. S. Jecker. 1995. *Wrong Medicine: Doctors, Patients and Futile Treatment.* Baltimore: Johns Hopkins University Press.

Weiner, J. P., B. H. Starfield, D. M. Steinwachs, and L. M. Mumford. 1991. "Development and Application of a Population-Oriented Measure of Ambulatory Care Case-Mix." *Medical Care* 29 (5): 452–72.

Weiner, J. P., A. Dobson, S. L. Maxwell, L. Coleman, B. H. Starfield, and G. E. Anderson. 1996. "Risk-Adjusted Medicare Capitation Rates Using Ambulatory and Inpatient Diagnoses." *Health Care Financing Review* 17 (3): 77–100.

Wennberg, J. E. 1998. "Variation in the Delivery of Health Care: The Stakes Are High." *Annals of Internal Medicine* 128 (10): 866–68.

Medicare Consumer Information and Risk Selection

Mark Merlis[1]

Because of limitations in Medicare's covered benefits, most beneficiaries seek supplemental insurance. They can choose from conventional Medigap plans, HMOs that contract with the Medicare
program, and, with the enactment of the Balanced Budget Act (BBA) of
1997, a variety of new managed care and fee-for-service alternatives collectively known as Medicare+Choice.

Currently, HMOs enjoy significant favorable selection and, as discussed
in Chapter 2, Medicare's payment system provides incentives to HMOs to
avoid enrolling high-risk beneficiaries. Some of the new options established
by the BBA may carry even greater potential for selection. The decisions
that beneficiaries will face will grow steadily more complicated and will
require them to assess the costs and benefits of different options, along with
delivery system restrictions and quality of care. To date, however, beneficiaries have had little access to clear and reliable comparisons of even the
most basic features of the choices available to them.

Improved consumer information could play a role in a broader strategy
to reduce selection bias. The BBA establishes an annual coordinated open
enrollment during which beneficiaries will have an opportunity to choose
from among Medicare+Choice plans available in their area (see Chapter 5).
HCFA is directed to conduct a national educational and publicity campaign

before each open enrollment period, with the costs to be defrayed through users' fees to be assessed on Medicare+Choice plans.[2] The new resources made available—up to $200 million in fiscal 1998, declining to $100 million for fiscal 2000 and later years—present an important opportunity for improving the information and enrollment process.

This chapter reviews the options available to beneficiaries and the kinds of information they now receive about those options. It then considers ways to improve the content of that information, to better regulate the information furnished to beneficiaries by health plans, and to develop alternative methods of communicating with beneficiaries. Finally, it tries to assess the likelihood that these measures will significantly affect selection bias.

MEDICARE OPTIONS

While the Medicare program was modeled on typical private health insurance plans at the time of its enactment in 1965, its benefits are now significantly less generous than those typically offered to private employee groups. Medicare imposes substantial cost-sharing for most of the services it covers and has no catastrophic limit on out-of-pocket costs. In 1995, Medicare paid 84.9 percent of costs for covered services; the remaining 15.1 percent was paid by beneficiaries (or by their supplemental coverage) in the form of required deductibles, coinsurance, and balance billing by providers (United States House of Representatives, Committee on Ways and Means 1996).[3] In addition, the program omits entirely such important services as outpatient prescription drugs. As a result, most beneficiaries obtain some form of supplemental coverage.

Table 4.1 shows sources of coverage for elderly and disabled non-institutionalized Medicare beneficiaries by income level in 1996. As the table indicates, 11 percent of beneficiaries rely on Medicaid to supplement Medicare, while 28 percent rely solely on retiree benefits from their former employers. These two groups, accounting for nearly two out of five beneficiaries, have a limited choice of supplemental plan. Most dually eligible Medicare/Medicaid beneficiaries remain in fee-for-service, although some states are moving to managed care for this population. Beneficiaries with retiree coverage may or may not be offered multiple options; in any event, the options available to them are selected by their former employers. These groups will not be addressed in this chapter; instead it will focus on the supplemental coverage choices available to beneficiaries who either purchase their own supplements on an individual basis or go without supplemental coverage. It should be noted, however, that the pool of all such beneficiaries will remain a subset of the total Medicare population, differing in unmeasured ways from dual eligibles and retirees. Even if there were no

Table 4.1 Sources of Supplemental Coverage, Elderly and Disabled Medicare Enrollees by Income Level Relative to the Poverty Line, 1996

	Under 100%		100–199%		200% or More		Total	
	Number	Percent	Number	Percent	Number	Percent	Number	Percent
Total Medicare	4,596	100.0%	10,687	100.0%	19,918	100.0%	35,201	100.0%
Medicare only	1,638	35.6	3,658	34.2	4,242	21.3	9,539	27.1
Medicare plus:								
Private supplement	665	14.5	3,215	30.1	5,589	28.1	9,468	26.9
Employer coverage	360	7.8	1,793	16.8	7,585	38.1	9,738	27.7
Medicaid	1,693	36.8	1,248	11.7	769	3.9	3,710	10.5
2 or more supplements	240	5.2	773	7.2	1,733	8.7	2,746	7.8

Source: IHPS analysis of data from the March 1997 Current Population Survey.

Note: It is uncertain whether enrollees in Medicare HMOs report themselves as having Medicare only or as having a private supplement.

biased selection within the group of individual purchasers, the overall Medicare risk pool would remain fragmented, with uncertain budgetary effects.[4]

Under the current system, a Medicare beneficiary seeking individual coverage has two basic choices: fee-for-service Medicare plus a supplemental private Medigap plan, or enrollment under a Medicare risk contract with an HMO or competitive medical plan (CMP), which provides all Medicare covered services plus some supplemental benefits.[5]

The BBA has broadened the types of health plans that may be offered to Medicare beneficiaries. It establishes three types of Medicare+Choice plans[6]:

1. Coordinated care plans, which, in addition to traditional HMOs, may include point-of-service plans, provider-sponsored organizations, and preferred provider organizations (PPOs); all of these plans use provider networks, with varying degrees of restriction on the use of out-of-network providers.

2. Medical savings account (MSA) plans, which provide high-deductible coverage to beneficiaries choosing to establish medical savings accounts and which may or may not use restrictive provider networks.

3. Private fee-for-service plans, which must cover the services of any qualified provider, paying at Medicare rates or rates negotiated with providers.

Table 4.2 summarizes key differences among the available options, along with their expected effects on the risk level of enrollees selecting each option. As the table suggests, each option has some features likely to encourage (indicated as +) and others likely to discourage (indicated as −) enrollment of high-risk beneficiaries.

Guaranteed Issue and Community Rating

All Medicare+Choice options are subject to guaranteed issue and community rating requirements. Medigap carriers are not subject to rating limits (unless imposed by a particular state) and must offer guaranteed issue only under very limited circumstances. A 1996 survey by the General Accounting Office (GAO) found that 11 out of the 25 largest Medigap carriers used medical underwriting for all of their policies and another five used underwriting for some policies (most commonly, those including outpatient prescription drugs). Only three of the carriers offered both guaranteed issue and community rating for all of their policies (USGAO 1996b). It would be expected that, in areas where HMOs or other alternative plans are available, the plans would function as insurers of last resort, attracting the uninsurable beneficiaries who are unable to obtain conventional Medigap or who face unacceptably high premiums (for example, because of attained age).[7] It may be that they are in fact performing this role for some high-risk beneficiaries. However, the overall favorable selection experienced by HMOs suggests that the market disadvantage created for them by the guaranteed issue requirement is outweighed by other factors.

Cost Sharing

Some of the new Medicare+Choice options expose beneficiaries to significant financial risk. MSA plans can impose a deductible of up to $6,000; there will also now be high-deductible Medigap plans.[8] Enrollees in private fee-for-service plans could be subject to significant balance billing by providers. All of these plans would be expected to attract beneficiaries who have a very low expectation of using health services (or who are misinformed—a very important reason for strengthening consumer information).

Supplemental Benefit

Medicare+Choice plans have wide latitude in defining supplemental benefits and could tailor benefit packages to attract low-risk applicants. However, the ten original options available to Medigap carriers also afford considerable opportunity for selection. For example, 6 of the 25 carriers examined by GAO offered no plan with prescription drug coverage, perhaps the benefit most likely to attract high utilizers of medical care.

Choice of Provider

Coordinated care plans require or encourage use of limited provider networks; MSA plans could establish networks. It has long been thought that high utilizers of services are more likely to have established ties to specific providers and are therefore reluctant to shift to restrictive networks. This may be especially true for the elderly. Although they may find that their primary care physician is participating in one of the network options available to them, beneficiaries with chronic conditions or multiple system problems may have ties to several different physicians. It may be unlikely that they can find a single network that includes all of their usual sources of care.

The stark difference between Medigap plans and coordinated care plans on this dimension may be diminishing. On the one hand, Medigap carriers are increasingly offering PPO-like Medicare Select policies. Some of these may be almost as restrictive as HMOs (except that beneficiaries can still see any Medicare provider if they pay the full required Medicare deductibles and coinsurance). At the same time, Medicare HMOs are increasingly offering a point-of-service option; the BBA also establishes a PPO option.

Table 4.2 Features of Medicare Supplemental Coverage Options and Expected Effects (+/–/?) on Risk Level of Enrollees

	Medigap	HMO or Other Coordinated Care Plan	MSA	Private Fee-for-Service
Eligibility	For elderly, must usually guarantee issue only during first six months after beneficiary enrolls in Part B (see text for exceptions). No guaranteed issue for disabled. (–)	Must guarantee issue during designated open enrollment periods. (+)	Must guarantee issue during designated open enrollment periods. (+)	Must guarantee issue during designated open enrollment periods. (+)
Rating Restrictions	Rates may vary by age at the time the policy is first issued or by "attained" age—the enrollee's age at the time of each renewal. Rates may also vary according to whether the policy is or is not medically underwritten. (–)	No variation permitted by age or other factors. (+)	No variation permitted by age or other factors. (+)	No variation permitted by age or other factors. (+)
Cost Sharing	Varies from first-dollar coverage (+) to coverage of coinsurance only (–). BBA also creates high-deductible options. (–)	Generally only nominal copayments (+); higher charges for out-of-network use in plans offering this option (?).	May impose deductible as high as $6,000 in 1999. (–)	Beneficiary potentially subject to substantial balance billing by providers. (–)

Continued

Table 4.2 (continued)

	Medigap	HMO or Other Coordinated Care Plan	MSA	Private Fee-for-Service
Supplemental Benefits	Must offer one of 12 standard benefit packages. (?)	May offer any package approved by secretary. (?)	May offer any package except one reducing deductible. (?)	May offer any package approved by secretary. (?)
Choice of Providers	Conventional—unrestricted. (+) Medicare Select—may cover (or reduce) cost-sharing only for in-network services. Enrollee using non-network providers receives Medicare payment but may pay usual Medicare cost-sharing. (−)	Traditional HMO or similar plan—payment available only for in-network services, except in emergency. (−) Point of service or PPO—some payment available for out-of-network services. (−) In both cases, enrollee waives Medicare payment for services not approved by plan.	May establish restricted network (−) or allow use of any provider (+).	Must allow use of any provider (+) but may have payment contracts with providers that would reduce beneficiary exposure to balance billing (?).

These new choices may gradually change the distribution of beneficiaries between Medigap carriers and HMOs. However, they will also make selection of a supplemental coverage source even more complex and confusing than it is today.

Price

Finally, there have been significant differences in the premiums charged to enrollees by Medigap and HMO plans. (Prices for the new options are not yet known.) In part because of greater efficiency and in part because of favorable selection, HMO costs for furnishing the basic Medicare services are less than the Medicare payments they receive. As a result, they can offer supplemental benefits for premiums well below those charged by conventional Medigap plans. In California, for example, the annual premium for Medigap Plan C offered through the American Association of Retired Persons was $893 in 1995, compared to an average annual premium of $117 for risk HMOs.[9] The national average annual HMO premium for basic coverage (at a minimum, waiver of all Medicare cost-sharing requirements except for nominal copayments) was $149.52 in February 1998, while 69 percent of plans charged no premium at all (HCFA 1998).

The effects of these rate differences on selection are uncertain. While substantial evidence exists that price influences the choice of health insurance plans, most available studies consider the effect of price on: (a) the decision to obtain coverage at all; (b) the decision to obtain additional benefits (for example, a high-option indemnity plan versus a low-option indemnity plan); or (c) selection among plans within a given plan type (for example, among competing HMOs).[10] One study that included plan type—differentiating between fee-for-service and IPA plans on the one hand and staff/group model HMOs on the other—found that year-to-year price changes would lead enrollees to switch from one plan to another within one of the two types but were less likely to induce enrollees to change plan type (Feldman et al. 1989).[11] These results would suggest that price alone may not be decisive for beneficiaries—whether sick or the "worried well"—who are reluctant to enter restrictive systems for other reasons.

It is intuitively likely that price would carry greater weight for lower income beneficiaries. Table 4.3 shows Medicare HMO penetration by annual income in 1993. The lowest and highest income beneficiaries were least likely to enroll in HMOs. Very low income beneficiaries who obtain supplemental coverage through Medicaid at no cost have less incentive than those just above Medicaid levels to join HMOs. High-income beneficiaries are more likely to have access to retiree benefits; those who do not can afford to pay higher premiums for less restrictive arrangements. HMO

Table 4.3   Estimated Medicare HMO Penetration by
Income, 1993

Annual Income	HMO Penetration
$5,000 or less	5.7%
$5,000–10,000	4.9
$10,000–15,000	7.3
$15,000–25,000	8.4
$25,000–50,000	7.5
over $50,000	4.1

Source: Calculated from Health Care Financing Administration. 1996. *Profiles of Medicare.*
Baltimore, Chart MC-14.

enrollment peaks among beneficiaries who are above poverty but who have limited discretionary income. While further investigation is obviously needed, this would suggest that, for modest-income beneficiaries, the financial advantages of HMOs outweigh concerns about their negative features. At higher income levels, people can afford to give non-price factors more weight in their decisions. These non-price factors—especially reluctance to switch physicians and concern about HMO limitations on access to specialist services—are likely to discourage high-risk people more than low service users, and so one would expect greater HMO favorable selection as income and the ability to pay the higher price of Medigap rises.

It is uncertain how the BBA will affect the relative weight of price and other factors that influence beneficiary choice. The BBA restricts growth in Medicare's capitation payments to HMOs and other Medicare+Choice plans to levels below expected growth in the fee-for-service sector. This may mean that HMOs will have to increase the premiums they charge enrollees for supplemental benefits. Second, payment for HMOs and other Medicare+Choice plans will gradually shift from area-specific rates to a national rate that will be adjusted for local input costs but not for local practice patterns. Plans in historically high-cost areas will see payment reductions that, again, may lead to higher charges or reduced benefits for enrollees. On the other hand, plans in historically low-cost areas will receive higher Medicare payments; they will be able to offer lower premiums or enhanced benefits to enrollees. The overall effect of the BBA on plan prices remains to be seen.

Nor is the potential effect of the introduction of new Medicare+Choice options clear. However, initially they will probably enter the choice set of a limited number of Medicare beneficiaries. The MSA option will be available only to one percent of beneficiaries on a time-limited demonstration basis. It is not yet possible to predict exactly what form private fee-for-service plans may take or how commonly they will be offered. For now, most beneficiaries will probably continue to face a basic choice between fee-for-service with or without Medigap and HMOs or other coordinated care plans; the remainder of this chapter will generally focus on that choice and on the continuing problem of favorable selection into HMOs.

The list of possible factors promoting favorable selection was discussed at length in Chapter 2. Three factors are particularly relevant to the discussion in this chapter:

- HMOs may be targeting low-risk enrollees deliberately, through selective marketing, benefit design, or other means.
- Beneficiaries are enrolled in the fee-for-service program by default and may remain there through inertia or because they are not aware of the other options available to them. This may affect particularly people who are very frail, housebound, or very old.
- The aversion of beneficiaries—especially high users of care—to managed care, because of concerns about access and quality, may be sufficient to outweigh the other apparent advantages of HMOs.

Various market reforms (discussed in Chapters 5 and 6) may change the impact of some of these factors. However, measures that directly address the factors militating against managed care enrollment by high-risk beneficiaries would have a more direct effect and greater likelihood of success in reducing selection bias. Possible steps include:

- preventing deliberate risk selection by health plans by stronger regulation (or elimination) of their direct marketing efforts;
- assuring that all beneficiaries fully understand their coverage options and the advantages and disadvantages of each; and
- providing information that will reduce beneficiary concern or modify preconceptions about managed care.

All of these steps involve information: ensuring that beneficiaries have access to reliable, unbiased, and comprehensible comparisons of their supplemental coverage options.

CURRENT INFORMATION FOR MEDICARE BENEFICIARIES AND ITS REGULATION

Beneficiaries learn about their coverage options through marketing efforts by health plans and Medigap carriers and through informational efforts by HCFA itself. They may also receive information from seniors' organizations, such as the American Association of Retired Persons, or from groups such as Consumers Union. While these third-party resources may be important to many beneficiaries, there is no systematic information about them, and they will not be addressed here.

HMO Marketing

HMOs generally market through their employed representatives and de-velop their own informational materials for prospective enrollees. HCFA places some restrictions on the activities of HMO representatives and requires that brochures, advertisements, and other marketing materials be reviewed in advance.[12] In addition, some states have licensure programs for HMO representatives comparable to those for other insurance agents or brokers.

HCFA review of marketing materials

HCFA must approve in advance all marketing materials, including adver-tisements, promotional material, information for prospective enrollees, and communications with current enrollees. Review covers any material tar-geted at Medicare beneficiaries as well as more general materials that in-clude any mention of Medicare. HCFA's guidelines for the content of mate-rials include numerous items that must be included, as well as certain kinds of statements that may not be made. The following are key points in the guidelines potentially relevant to risk selection.

Materials must:

- indicate that all Medicare beneficiaries (not just the elderly) are eligible to join and that the HMO may not discriminate by health status;
- explain the HMO's supplemental benefits, premiums, and cost-shar-ing requirements;
- explain how to obtain services, with special emphasis on clarifying network restrictions, gatekeeper and prior authorization requirements, and exceptions for emergency and out-of-area care;
- explain disenrollment procedures and explain that enrollment may be terminated if the HMO's Medicare contract is terminated;
- warn beneficiaries that if they give up their Medigap coverage, they may not be able to obtain it again if they disenroll from the HMO; and
- include a listing of contracting providers.

Materials may not:

- suggest that HCFA has recommended or endorsed the plan;
- make inaccurate statements about Medicare's benefits or the plan's benefits; or
- imply perpetual coverage.

HCFA restrictions on representatives

Medicare marketing representatives are usually HMO employees. (HCFA "strongly discourages" but does not prohibit the use of independent agents.)

HCFA suggests that Medicare representatives should meet the same standards the HMO uses for its commercial representatives.

The following restrictions apply to marketing activities:

- Representatives are not permitted to engage in door-to-door marketing. However, there are no restrictions on their contact with beneficiaries who have expressed an interest in learning more about the HMO—for example, by responding to a mailing or a telephone solicitation.
- Gifts or payments as an inducement to enroll (or to refer other beneficiaries for enrollment) are prohibited (except gifts of nominal value provided whether or not the beneficiary enrolls). Rebates or other rewards for reduced utilization are also prohibited.

HMOs are encouraged to develop systems to assure that their representatives are providing accurate information, particularly on benefits and network restrictions. Suggested measures include:

- an enrollment verification system to confirm that new Medicare applicants understand the HMO's restrictions before enrolling;
- a system for tracking disenrollment rates by representative, to identify specific representatives who may be providing inadequate information; and
- a compensation system for representatives that rewards sustained retention of enrollees rather than simple volume.

Finally, HCFA "strongly discourages" but does not prohibit the use of affiliated physicians or other providers as marketing agents for HMOs/CMPs. (The issue of provider marketing is discussed further below.)

Medigap Marketing

Medigap policies, like other insurance in the individual market, may be sold by the insurer's own employees or by outside agents and brokers. Oversight of Medigap marketing is chiefly left to the states. States approve policies and informational materials and require licensure for independent agents.

Agent licensure

Over the years states have established licensing requirements for those marketing or selling insurance. All states require that individuals pass a written exam or complete an approved course of study in order to be licensed as agents. However, state licensing requirements vary widely in the rigor of their training and examination programs. Most state licenses permit the sale of a range of different types of insurance (e.g., life, health, accidental death and dismemberment). Licenses are typically renewed annually.

The actual effect of licensure varies from state to state. In the minimalist states, licensure acts largely as a mechanism to sanction retrospectively those who undertake unethical or otherwise unacceptable business practices. Such enforcement generally occurs as a result of customer complaints to the state insurance department. In most cases states sanction agents through fines. In more serious or repeated cases agents may have their license revoked. For example, a state may revoke an agent's license if he or she commits fraud or provides a rebate to customers (such as a cut of the agent's commission). More active states view licensing as an opportunity to actively oversee market conduct and to educate and test individuals for the basic knowledge and character deemed necessary to market or sell insurance.

Although many states make a distinction between agents and brokers, there are no clear and common definitions. The licensing and educational requirements for agents and brokers are often similar or identical. Perhaps the most important difference between an agent and a broker is that an agent generally has contractual relationships with one or more health plans while brokers have a contractual relationship with the purchaser. In addition, brokers deal with many different insurers or plans while agents often have relationships with only one or a small number of insurers.[13] However, both agents and brokers typically receive remuneration from the insurer or plan.

Federal requirements

Limited federal requirements for Medigap marketing also exist, largely focused on eliminating sales practices that may frighten elderly people into purchasing multiple, duplicative Medigap policies.[14] Agents are now required to ascertain whether an individual already has supplemental coverage (including Medicaid) and may not sell a policy unless the beneficiary intends to terminate existing coverage and replace it with the new policy.

Other federal requirements are as follows:

- Agents must inform beneficiaries of the availability of state-managed information, counseling, and assistance (ICA) programs (see the discussion of these programs in the next section).
- Insurers must provide an outline of coverage that uses uniform language and format to facilitate comparison among Medigap policies and comparison with Medicare benefits.
- Agents may not claim to be acting under the authority of or in association with Medicare or other federal agencies.
- Advertising must be reviewed or approved by the state (to the extent required under state law).

Potential for Abuse Under the Current System

The heavy reliance on health plans and carriers to provide beneficiaries with information about their coverage options presents numerous opportunities for misinforming beneficiaries or for deliberately screening out high-risk applicants. The following discussion is confined to concerns raised by HMO marketing practices. Because Medigap carriers can simply deny coverage to high-risk applicants (after the six-month enrollment window at age 65, or except in special circumstances described earlier), they have less reason to rely on more subtle risk selection techniques. The major concern in Medigap regulation has therefore been the sale of unnecessary coverage. If Medigap carriers were required to guarantee issue and use community rating, they might face the same incentives now faced by HMOs, with a similar potential for abuse.[15]

Basic marketing strategies

Current oversight of HMO marketing deals largely with practices that may induce enrollees to join HMOs without fully understanding the consequences of enrollment. For example, review guidelines for marketing materials put the greatest emphasis on ensuring that provider restrictions and authorization requirements are fully and prominently explained. While this information is obviously essential, little attention is paid to practices that *discourage* enrollment by high-risk beneficiaries.

This emphasis presumably stems from the fact that inadequately informed enrollees are a major source of complaints, grievances, and disenrollment. In addition, HCFA's focus may derive from experiences under Medicaid in the 1970s and Medicare in the 1980s, when some organizations pursued strategies of rapidly and aggressively enrolling as many beneficiaries as possible. Some organizations may still pursue this strategy, and continued scrutiny is appropriate. However, the potential for selection arises when an HMO chooses to concern itself with the characteristics of enrollees, not merely with the number of enrollees it attracts.

In the health insurance industry generally, there are competing objectives that may be thought of as representing an ongoing tension between the marketing and actuarial departments. The marketing department seeks enrollment growth. An individual marketing representative's performance is measured in terms of meeting or exceeding a monthly or yearly quota of new sales. The representative has a strong incentive to achieve a quick sale, even at the price of misinforming or under-informing the client, so as to be free to move on to the next potential client. From the perspective of the actuarial department, on the other hand, high volume is only good news if it is "high quality"—the industry's traditional term for policyholders who can be expected to have favorable claims experience.

This tension has traditionally been resolved through underwriting: the representative brings in the maximum number of possible applicants, and the underwriting department winnows out those presenting high risk. As Medicare HMOs cannot engage in underwriting, they must balance the conflicting objectives of volume and "quality" within the marketing process itself. The marketing department may therefore be evaluated on its ability to screen out undesirable applicants, as well as on the total number of applications it generates.

Direct beneficiary contact

Direct contact between HMO representatives and Medicare beneficiaries gives the HMO an opportunity to assess the risk level presented by the beneficiary. Representatives can market less vigorously to—or even discourage enrollment by—potentially high-cost applicants. Representatives may be able to visually identify seriously ill beneficiaries or ascertain their health status in a few simple questions. In turn, the questions asked by a beneficiary may signal a potential for high utilization. For example, a beneficiary may inquire about the availability of a particular specialty service or about the inclusion of a high-cost drug in the HMO's formulary. In either case, the representative need not actually refuse to enroll the beneficiary, which is prohibited. He or she can simply prematurely conclude a marketing presentation, or suggest that the HMO may not be the right coverage choice for that beneficiary. The opportunities for informal screening are not limited to face-to-face meetings between representatives and beneficiaries. Similar effects can be achieved even when HMO personnel are simply responding to telephone inquiries about the HMO's coverage or services.

There is no empirical evidence, beyond anecdotes, that HMOs actively discourage individual high-risk applicants. For reasons discussed below, such evidence would be difficult to collect. However, the opportunities for selection through direct beneficiary contact are real and the financial rewards substantial; it would be imprudent to assume that no organization will engage in this practice, especially when it violates no current rule.

Targeted marketing

HMOs' marketing efforts may be targeted to specific populations that are healthier than average. HCFA explicitly forbids marketing restricted to high-income areas, or efforts to target newly eligible beneficiaries. However, routine practices permitted by HCFA allow considerable room for selection. For example, group presentations at senior centers or similar venues necessarily reach only those beneficiaries who are active and mobile. Even promotions aimed at the entire elderly population miss the non-elderly disabled).

Targeting may also be more subtle. For example, a common marketing strategy is to make the target audience identify closely with the marketing piece. An HMO may develop marketing brochures, billboards, and television ads that depict healthy and active elderly people and avoid depictions of people receiving medical services, with the implication that the HMO is a club that sick people need not join.

Marketing by providers

Physicians or other providers who participate in multiple plans, or in both an HMO and fee-for-service Medicare, have extensive health information about their existing patients and clear incentives to steer them to the plan that will provide the best compensation. For example, a physician paid by a plan on a capitated basis may wish to have low-risk patients in that plan and leave higher utilizers in Medicare fee-for-service. Incentives are likely to grow more complex if providers are also involved in organizing provider-sponsored organizations or have participation agreements with private fee-for-service plans.

Even in the absence of incentives to steer patients, physicians may still influence patients' coverage decisions. They may, for example, advise patients with multi-system problems to avoid plans with a limited choice of specialists. As was noted earlier, HCFA "discourages" but does not prohibit provider marketing. Guidance issued in August 1997 places a number of restrictions on provider activities (HCFA 1997). Providers may distribute marketing materials but may not make comparisons among plans or accept enrollment applications; if they send mailings to beneficiaries, they are not allowed to screen for health status; if they give lists of Medicare-eligible patients to health plans, the lists must be complete and must not include information on age or health status. While these rules may limit abuse in systematic marketing efforts by providers, compliance may be difficult to monitor, and opportunities will remain for physicians to offer informal guidance to their patients.

The HMO itself has health information about its current enrollees. An insurer that offers both a risk HMO product and a Medicare Select plan using the same network could encourage some enrollees to shift from one to the other. Steering may be especially feasible for HMO enrollees who are turning 65 and are eligible for conversion from employer-sponsored or individual enrollment to Medicare status. While the HMO may not deny such a conversion, it could suggest to selected newly eligible beneficiaries that they would be better served under their new Medicare fee-for-service benefit.

As in the case of direct beneficiary contact, there is no hard evidence of systematic steering of current patients by providers or HMOs. Again, however, there are clear opportunities for abusive practices and significant financial incentives to engage in them. Concerns about this possibility will only be heightened as Medicare begins to contract directly with provider-sponsored organizations that also maintain a fee-for-service operation.

Misplaced emphasis

An HMO's marketing materials and direct presentations may be entirely accurate but may emphasize features of the plan that are of potential interest to healthy beneficiaries—such as preventive services—and de-emphasize features likely to attract sicker beneficiaries—such as the availability of specialized treatment programs for high-cost conditions. Again, the opportunities for selective emphasis are greatest in face-to-face presentations. For example, presentations to beneficiaries perceived as high-risk may be especially emphatic about the restrictions entailed by HMO enrollment.

HCFA Initiatives on Beneficiary Information

HCFA has made efforts to improve the information available to beneficiaries on coverage options and to develop alternatives to direct plan marketing. The following is an overview of current information programs.

HCFA publications

HCFA has a number of publications that include information about HMOs and other coverage options. Some of these are furnished to all beneficiaries; others are available on request, through counseling programs, and on the Internet. Relevant consumer publications include:

- the *Medicare Handbook*, which summarizes Medicare benefits, rights, and obligations, and answers frequently asked questions;
- the *Guide to Health Insurance for People with Medicare*, which explains how to choose a Medigap plan and includes information on the HMO option;
- *Medicare Managed Care*, which explains the difference between fee-for-service and HMOs and describes HMO enrollment; and
- *Know Your Rights*, a Medicare Beneficiary Advisory Bulletin on HMOs, jointly developed by HCFA and the Office of the Inspector General.

HCFA's Internet site includes these publications (www.medicare.gov/ comparison). The site now has a feature called Medicare Compare that provides comparative information about individual health plans, costs, premiums, and services provided, as well as information on enrollment and disenrollment rules, a glossary of terms, and questions and answers.

Information, counseling, and advocacy programs[16]

To assist Medicare beneficiaries in making decisions regarding their health insurance coverage, the Omnibus Budget Reconciliation Act (OBRA) of

1990 established federally funded, state-managed information, counseling, and assistance (ICA) programs. In addition to receiving basic funding for ICA programs, states with Medicare HMOs are provided additional funds to promote understanding of managed care plan options. ICA programs are administered primarily through state departments on aging (two-thirds) or departments of insurance (one-third). An estimated three-fourths of all counties nationwide have at least one local counseling site, staffed by a combination of paid staff and an estimated 10,500 state-trained older adult volunteers who provide the bulk of services.

ICA programs are generally responsible for providing information on a variety of different topics, including information about Medicare in general, supplemental insurance products, long-term care insurance, managed care plans, and eligibility for Medicaid and other public programs. Each state is responsible for defining its own program. In addition, some states have also developed a spectrum of senior information and counseling services financed with state funds. California, for example, funds its counseling programs through an earmarked portion of insurance agent and broker licensure fees.

Medicare beneficiaries are served through individual face-to-face counseling, telephone consultation, group presentations, and written materials. ICAs can also help beneficiaries complete claims forms and file appeals. Programs in half of the states have developed consumer guidebooks. Many states have also developed written pamphlets and materials (e.g., comparability charts) to better explain features of Medicare managed care plans.

HCFA works closely with ICA programs through the national ICA Steering Committee and Resource Center to develop and provide information on managed care. Most recently HCFA has developed an ICA training module and video containing information on the basics of managed care, as well as case studies, for use by all ICA programs for their volunteer orientation and training programs.[17]

In an early year of operation, ICA programs served approximately 192,212 individuals via phone or one-to-one counseling (April 1, 1993–March 31, 1994). This figure represented not quite one percent of elderly Medicare beneficiaries. In addition, more than 400,000 people participated in a presentation or seminar. Only 5 percent of the total health insurance issues raised during counseling encounters dealt with managed care questions, although states with a high level of managed care penetration, such as California, Massachusetts, and Oregon, had higher percentages.

An evaluation of the first year of ICA programs' experience reported that it provides a valued service and has attracted committed volunteers and in-kind support, although evaluators recommended increased publicity and outreach and more standardized data collection and sharing of materials.

However, neither the ICA program evaluation nor the few assessments of earlier programs for providing health insurance information to Medicare beneficiaries has demonstrated a clear effect on knowledge, attitudes, or decision-making.

Use of enrollment brokers

HCFA is also planning to test the use of a third-party open enrollment broker as a tool to provide beneficiaries with education about their Medicare coverage options, both fee-for-service and managed care, and to provide assistance in making the coverage choice that best meets their needs. (Third-party brokers have been used extensively by state Medicaid agencies; their experience is discussed later in this chapter.) This test was originally planned as part of the Competitive Pricing Demonstration project. The BBA authorizes a distinct enrollment broker demonstration that must not be combined with any other demonstration. Issues surrounding the use of a broker will be discussed further below.

Information Requirements Under the BBA

Under the BBA, the Secretary for Health and Human Services will be required to mail the following information to beneficiaries before the start of each annual open enrollment period:

- general information, including a description of benefits under the Medicare fee-for-service program, a discussion of Medigap and Medicare select, an explanation of the Medicare+Choice enrollment process, and information on enrollee rights and the possibility and consequences of contract termination by a Medicare+ Choice plan;
- a comparative listing of Medicare+Choice plans available in the area, including service area, premiums, supplemental benefits, cost-sharing and out-of-pocket limits, and network restrictions, including restrictions on the ability to select from among providers within the network; and
- "to the extent available," quality and performance indicators for plans, including comparisons with the performance of the Medicare fee-for-service program on the same indicators. These indicators include disenrollment rates, satisfaction information, information on health outcomes, and the plan's record of compliance with Medicare requirements.

In addition to conducting the annual mailing, the secretary must maintain a toll-free number for inquiries about Medicare+Choice options and continue offering plan comparisons on an Internet site. All of these activities may be contracted out.

Some additional information is not required to be provided by the secretary (although the secretary has the statutory authority to include it in the annual mailing) but must be disclosed by the Medicare+Choice organization itself at the request of a beneficiary. This includes the organization's utilization control methods, physician incentive plans, and record of grievances and appeals of service denials.

WHAT DO BENEFICIARIES NEED TO KNOW?

The BBA has established a somewhat more structured multiple choice system for Medicare beneficiaries—though with the crucial omission of Medigap plans from the structure—and has provided HCFA with resources and authority to inform beneficiaries about their choices under the new system. This section and the next will discuss some of the key issues in designing an information program, including what beneficiaries need to be told and who should tell it to them.

Barriers to Choice

Much of what is known about the role of consumer information in health plan choice stems from experience in the private market and the Medicaid program. While the following discussion draws on that experience, some features of the Medicare program and population may limit the applicability of lessons learned in other sectors.

Individual enrollment

Medicare beneficiaries enter the supplemental coverage market as individual purchasers and are harder to reach than people who obtain coverage in a group environment.

It may be difficult to ensure that all beneficiaries receive and understand information about their coverage options, and even more difficult to ensure that they all actively select from among those options. The experience of state Medicaid programs that have mandated HMO enrollment by certain Medicaid populations is instructive. In 1996, the GAO studied the programs in four states that made substantial efforts to educate beneficiaries about their health plan choices. In each state, a significant proportion of beneficiaries did not choose among the available plans and had to be assigned to a plan by the state. Assignment rates ranged from 12 percent in Minnesota to as high as 41 percent in Ohio (USGAO 1996a).

It may be at least as difficult to induce Medicare beneficiaries to make a rational choice among health plans. Even those with no cognitive disability may have had little experience in choosing among health plans during their working life. Moreover, those who have the greatest difficulty in understanding their options and making a selection may also be the highest risk enrollees.

Fee-for-service default

Medicare beneficiaries are enrolled by default in the fee-for-service system and must actively choose to switch to a Medicare+Choice plan. While there are many multiple choice programs, it is now rare for participants' options to be presented in this fashion. (Those Medicaid programs that still offer voluntary HMO enrollment are the one other major setting in which enrollees who fail to make a selection are automatically assigned to the fee-for-service plan.) In addition, of course, the default plan under Medicare is not just one on a list of competing plans, as when a federal employee is given a choice of Blue Cross/Blue Shield, various HMOs, and so on. Medicare is *Medicare*, a program that—whatever the status of the trust funds—is backed by the faith and credit of the United States government. All other plans are likely to be perceived as *not Medicare*. Some beneficiaries may consider the choice between fee-for-service and an HMO not as a choice about how to receive Medicare benefits but as a choice about whether to receive Medicare or some other health insurance.

The default status of fee-for-service contributes to what is likely to be a major factor in beneficiary self-selection: inertia. People who are not seriously dissatisfied with their current coverage may be reluctant to change that coverage even if better-priced or otherwise more advantageous options are available. This tendency may be even greater among elderly people. The GAO study of Medigap coverage cited earlier found that 99 percent of beneficiaries who had private plans in 1991 and were still alive in 1994 had the same plan in 1994 (USGAO 1996a). The loyalty of elderly people to their current coverage is further suggested by the experience of the Federal Employees Health Benefits Program (FEHBP) in the late 1980s, when one of the two government-wide indemnity plans still available dropped out of the program. Although participants were told that they needed to select a new plan from among the other FEHBP options, many annuitants failed or even actively refused to do so; ultimately they were assigned to the remaining indemnity plan.

The private sector has had some experience with campaigns to make participants in multiple choice systems aware that they have a choice of health plans and motivate them to make a careful and thoughtful choice. Beneficiaries' interest in getting information—as evidenced by how much time they will spend acquiring and understanding the information, how much of their attention is focused on the information, and how much time and attention they will give to getting information from other sources—can be enhanced by materials (both targeted and mass media) that contain key messages that resonate with beneficiaries' concerns. A typical appeal to a young employed population may be, "You want a health plan that works hard to provide high quality care for you and your family. New information is available to help you choose." Appropriate cognitive testing should be done to determine which similar messages may resonate best with Medicare beneficiaries.

Fee-for-service inertia may also be partially addressed through some clearer indication that HMOs and other alternatives are still Medicare. HCFA's current rules for HMO marketing materials prohibit any suggestion that HCFA has endorsed or recommended a plan. Yet HCFA does make decisions with respect to plans: HMOs and CMPs must meet a long list of standards before entering into a contract and are subject to periodic monitoring thereafter. While there may be debate over the methods or adequacy of current HMO oversight, HCFA is engaged in a form of selective contracting. Every plan available has been found to be good enough. It may be useful for beneficiaries to know this and to know, at least in general terms, what steps HCFA went through in determining that an organization was eligible. Some beneficiaries may wonder, for example, "Could this plan go out of business without paying my bills?" They might be reassured to learn that HCFA has required some basic assurances against insolvency. The distinction between recommendation and mere approval is a subtle one, and a way must be found of conveying it without suggesting that all approved plans are equally good choices. Still, beneficiaries should know that every plan has met some basic tests.

Promoting Basic System Understanding

Medicare beneficiaries make not one but three health plan choices:

1. whether to obtain supplemental coverage at all;
2. whether to choose Medigap or some type of Medicare+Choice plan; and
3. which individual carrier or plan to select.

The gaps in Medicare coverage expose beneficiaries to substantial risk. One would expect that most beneficiaries who forego supplemental coverage do so because they cannot find affordable coverage. However, as Table 4.1 shows, even some higher income beneficiaries lack supplemental coverage. Some of these may be uninsurable. Others may anticipate little need for medical care. Still others may be unaware of the limits of Medicare coverage and the need for a supplement. The existence of the group of non-purchasers further fragments the risk pool. It also suggests that one of the first roles of consumer information efforts may be to promote better understanding of the Medicare program itself.

Consumers generally and older adults in particular have a low level of knowledge of health insurance and Medicare coverage (Sofaer 1995). As a result, a consistent finding in studies of the information needs of Medicare beneficiaries is that newly enrolled beneficiaries, as well as some longer-term beneficiaries, need basic information about the Medicare program in general, its coverage gaps, and supplemental coverage options (Gibbs 1995).

Beneficiaries also have a limited understanding of managed care. Studies have shown that while awareness of HMOs has increased among Medicare beneficiaries in recent years and the federal government has funded a number of programs designed to educate beneficiaries regarding Medicare HMOs, beneficiaries nevertheless often exhibit low levels of knowledge about HMO plans and confusion or misunderstanding about the principles of managed care (Sofaer 1995). This is consistent with findings relating to consumers of all ages in the private sector. A national survey conducted in 1995 found that a high percentage of Americans do not understand the basic elements of health plans; for example, 67 percent said that they do not have a good understanding of the differences between traditional fee-for-service and managed care plans (Isaacs 1996).

The proliferation of delivery models that are more restrictive than Medicare fee-for-service but less restrictive than traditional HMOs may make managed care less threatening to high-risk beneficiaries, but they also dramatically complicate the difficulties of understanding the choices available. Plans will have different rules on the role of gatekeepers, when and at what cost unauthorized or out-of-network specialty services may be obtained, and so on. Beneficiaries will need to assess tradeoffs between various levels of freedom of choice and of financial exposure; even in a single plan, those tradeoffs may vary according to patterns of utilization.

Beneficiaries will also need some way of assessing different benefit packages. Many successful consumer choice initiatives have moved toward standardized benefits across plans, enabling participants to compare plans on two dimensions: premium cost and quality (how the consumer defines quality is considered below). The BBA's failure to standardize benefits means that beneficiaries must compare plans on a third—and especially confusing—dimension. It may be possible to furnish comparative information on the average actuarial value of different benefit packages. However, averages cannot reflect the value of a package to participants with different needs.

An alternative may be to construct healthcare scenarios and show what the consumer would have to pay under the various plans. For example, here is what a participant requiring a coronary bypass would typically pay under Plan A, Plan B; here is what a participant requiring maintenance medications would pay; and so on. Illustrations of this kind have appeared in the guidebooks to federal employee health plans published by Washington Consumer Checkbook. Of course, the more scenarios that are provided, the more readily consumers with different needs can self-select into the plans offering them the most favorable cost structure. The selection would, however, be *informed* selection. As will be suggested at the conclusion of this chapter, the goal of reducing selection bias must be balanced against the goal of helping beneficiaries choose what is right for them.

Comparative Plan Information

Assuming that beneficiaries can be motivated to think carefully about their health plan choices and have absorbed basic information about benefits and delivery structures, they will then be ready to consider comparative information about individual plans.

There are currently only limited data on how Medicare beneficiaries make decisions to join Medicare plans and what information they need to support these decisions (Institute of Medicine 1996). Studies have attempted to ascertain what information beneficiaries "want," "need," identify as "of interest," or rate as "important." However, it is not necessarily the case that items of information so identified actually play a key role in determining selection of health coverage. An abundance of data can potentially be provided to consumers under the heading of consumer information, but it may actually have little bearing on their decision-making processes.

In an examination of consumer plan-switching behavior, David Mechanic noted that consumers tend to base their decisions on a small number of salient criteria rather than on all the measures they would rate as "important" (1989). Similarly, the Office of Technology Assessment's Expert Advisory Panel on Quality of Medical Care Information for Consumers concluded in its 1988 review of social sciences literature about how individuals make choices that:

> To more effectively inform consumers about the quality of providers' care, limiting information to only a few indicators of quality will probably be necessary. People can consider only a few items at any one time. Information is processed as a unit or chunk—a person's processing capacity has been estimated as being anywhere from four to seven chunks. (U.S. Congress, Office of Technology Assessment 1988)

This concept is relevant because the number and variety of measures of the quality of care and services delivered by managed care plans is growing at a remarkable rate. For Medicare plans, HCFA is already collecting the following data that could potentially be used in plan comparisons:

- *Performance measurements.* All Medicare managed care plans are required to report their performance on a standardized set of performance measures (the National Committee for Quality Assurance's HEDIS 3.0) on an annual basis. HCFA is also working with other groups, such as the Foundation for Accountability (FACCT) to develop and test alternative measures.

- *Survey of Medicare beneficiaries.* All managed care plans contracting with Medicare administer through an external vendor the Consumer Assessment of Health Plans Study (CAHPS) questionnaire. The survey results will provide HCFA with plan-specific information on how satisfied beneficiaries are with the care received and how beneficiaries assess health plan performance in such areas as provider communication and access to needed services.

- *Analysis of inquiries and complaints.* HCFA has a toll-free hotline known as the Beneficiary Inquiry Tracking System (BITS). From this automated system, HCFA aggregates and analyzes managed care inquiries and complaints received from beneficiaries and other concerned parties on subjects such as quality of care, enrollment/disenrollment, and bill payment problems.

- *Disenrollment data.* HCFA can track the number of disenrollments occurring on a periodic basis from each health plan.

- *Results of quality monitoring.* HCFA has information on the results of its ongoing quality monitoring activities (e.g., annual external quality reviews conducted by quality review and improvement organizations (QIOs), and periodic comprehensive monitoring of plan compliance with quality of care standards).

Additional measures could easily be added. The proliferation of measures has been so rapid that public and private efforts are under way simply to catalog and describe all available quality of care measures. One of these efforts, Project CONQUEST, has catalogued more than 53 separate measurement sets containing more than 1,100 quality of care measures.

Obviously there will have to be some basis for selecting which measures should actually be presented to consumers. One option is to develop a composite or aggregate measure that merges results on a number of performance indicators. However, decisions on which indicators to include and how to weight them are likely to be controversial, particularly if plan performance is not consistent across measures.

An alternative is to attempt to identify the measures Medicare beneficiaries themselves regard as important. Much of the research on this subject has relied on focus groups. The following is a summary of the findings of some key studies.

In 1995, on behalf of the Kaiser Family Foundation, Frederick/ Schneiders Inc. conducted 14 focus groups with Medicare beneficiaries (Frederick/Schneiders Inc. 1995). The focus groups were designed to explore the attitudes and experiences of Medicare beneficiaries in managed care plans and traditional fee-for-service, as well as experiences of adults aged 60–65 who were not yet Medicare beneficiaries but who would be shortly and thus would need to make decisions about Medicare coverage options.

Their findings underscored the fact that beneficiaries vary in their experiences and in their beliefs about and receptivity to managed care, and that these experiences and beliefs shape beneficiaries' desires for information about health plans. However, these focus groups did determine that ability to choose a specific practitioner is frequently an overarching determinant of health coverage selected: "Few consumers are motivated to change doctors in order to receive the benefits offered by HMOs." A related concern of beneficiaries includes the perceived quality of doctors' interactions with patients. Interpersonal issues were mentioned more frequently than clinical competence as a concern, but this should not be interpreted as indicating that interpersonal care is more important than clinical competence. It could indicate that clinical competence is assumed, while consumers' experience has led them to believe that attentive, respectful, and compassionate care should not be. Alternatively, Frederick/Schneiders concluded that the emphasis on the interpersonal may indicate beneficiaries' difficulty in evaluating technical competence; as a result, they focus on the aspect of patient-provider relationships that they do feel comfortable in evaluating. Cost and coverage ranked next highest as criteria for selecting the type of healthcare coverage.

Also in 1995, the National Committee for Quality Assurance (NCQA) conducted six focus groups to address the questions of how consumers:

- evaluate options and select plans;
- define and find quality of healthcare;
- rank factors such as cost, coverage, and choice of doctor in their coverage decisions;
- think about quality in selecting a health plan;
- identify and use information relevant to plan selection decisions;
- think about information being developed for consumers; and
- react to specific models of data presented. (National Committee for Quality Assurance 1995)

One of the focus groups was composed entirely of retired individuals. The findings of this focus group were consistent in some areas with those of other focus groups composed of younger (< 65 years of age) individuals.

Issues that consumers rated as most significant for their choice decisions were costs, coverage, and how plans worked. Ratings of satisfaction with care and quality of care were rated as less important.

The quality-of-care issues ranked most important by consumers were skills of the physician, including interpersonal communication and technical competence; access to care, especially in an emergency; reminders about preventive services such as Pap smears; and coverage for follow-up services such as physical therapy and rehabilitation.

Another 1995 analysis of information needs for consumer choice for HCFA that included Medicare beneficiaries as a targeted group also found that Medicare beneficiaries were concerned about access to their current primary care providers as well as specialists, providers' communication skills, benefits, and technical quality of care (Gibbs 1995).

In 1996, the NCQA conducted an additional five focus groups with Medicare beneficiaries; a sixth was held with family members who help make healthcare coverage decisions for Medicare beneficiaries (National Committee for Quality Assurance 1996). In these focus groups, quality-of-care measures (technical quality of care, patient satisfaction, and access to care) were presented alone. Information on cost, coverage, providers, and rules for obtaining care was not provided. When quality of care was presented to consumers in this way, the focus groups found that Medicare beneficiaries are interested in and appreciate receiving comparative information on measures of access, technical quality, and patient satisfaction, especially if it was on topics they found important and if the information was from a source they found trustworthy. Measures of ease of access to care and services (in contrast to measures of technical quality of care and patient satisfaction with care) were the measures that were most appreciated by focus group participants. Participants expressed strong interest in measures of ease of access to urgent, after hours, and emergency care. Participants also placed importance on being able to get to the right specialist, being able to choose and change doctors, and being able to see the same doctor on most visits.

In sum, beneficiaries appear to be chiefly interested in cost and choice of providers, then in access and interpersonal aspects of quality. Technical quality is of less importance, possibly because beneficiaries are skeptical about quality measurement at the plan level or do not find specific measures to be relevant to their concerns.

Helping Beneficiaries Use the Data

Beneficiaries require more than comparative information when choosing among plans. They also need help in sorting that information and identifying what is most important to them. No effort will be made here to summarize the growing body of literature on how consumers use information and make choices, but it may be useful to highlight a few key points.

Individuals use natural heuristics to process information and make complicated decisions. For example, they may apply one or more key criteria (such as cost or whether a given doctor is in the network) to narrow their options to a manageable number. Some focus on maximizing positive characteristics; others try to minimize negatives. In addition, people differ in their ability to evaluate various kinds of information (for example, quantitative versus graphic). It is important that consumer choice information accommodate a range of cognitive capacities and learning styles.

The source of information can be important. In general, beneficiaries are likely to consider information obtained from other consumers (both through formal surveys and informal interactions) as highly credible—along with information from their providers. Consumers are more likely to trust information about benefits and coverage that comes from health plans, but they are often skeptical of quality information provided by health plans unless it has been validated or presented by an objective third party.

Beneficiaries differ in their access and response to various information channels. The experience of employers who have worked with retirees, such as Southern California Edison, and other organizations that provide assistance and choice counseling to Medicare enrollees indicate that personal interactions—whether one-on-one or in group presentations—are very popular with many Medicare beneficiaries. Others may be more likely to respond to print or video, and a small but growing number of beneficiaries turn to the Internet for information.

Because motivation, salience, and ability vary from individual to individual, not all beneficiaries will be interested in the same level of detail. It is possible to provide access to different levels of detail through a process of *layering* information. An example of layered information about health plan quality could begin by presenting comparisons of overall plan performance, then presenting composites of performance on different dimensions of quality that aggregate a plan's scores on several individual measures related to that dimension, then perhaps allowing beneficiaries to review detailed information about each measure included in the composite if they choose.

Over time, there is hope of constructing information systems with built-in heuristics and extensive "decision support" (meaning systems that narrow the choices based on stated preferences or that result in evaluative judgments such as "these plans are the best fit for you"). Such systems could be used in face-to-face or telephone counseling or could be embodied in interactive computer programs. However, much further research will be required.

In addition, because some studies have suggested that key selection criteria for any individual may not be stable over time, systems to identify the best fit for any client should be developed with caution.

HOW CAN INFORMATION GIVEN TO BENEFICIARIES BE CONTROLLED BETTER?

Stronger Regulation of Plan Marketing Activities

As was suggested earlier, the heavy reliance on plans as sources of information for beneficiaries offers numerous opportunities for targeted marketing and possibly for more serious abuses, such as active discouragement of enrollment by beneficiaries perceived to be high risk. Because it is impossible to monitor every contact between a plan and a potential enrollee, it may be difficult to control—or even identify—practices of this kind. Even in the absence of any abuse, presentations by plan representatives are unlikely to be very helpful to beneficiaries seeking the best option from the multiplicity of choices that may soon be available in some areas. While a representative may be able to fairly compare his or her specific plan with fee-for-service Medicare, the beneficiary will not learn about the other choices available.

Ideally, it may be best to remove plans from the entire marketing and enrollment process, as some states have done under their Medicaid programs. Plans might be permitted to develop marketing materials under very careful oversight but would be prohibited from initiating any direct contact with potential enrollees. Instead, beneficiaries would obtain information from independent sources or neutral brokers. The possibility of developing these alternate conduits for information will be discussed further below.

As a practical matter, however, it is unlikely that plans will be removed from the marketing process in the near future. If alternate information sources are developed, they may be obliged to operate alongside continued plan marketing efforts. If so, at least some steps could be taken to reduce the opportunities for selection.

Training and licensure of representatives

Federal standards could be established for training and licensure of plans' employed representatives, comparable to state requirements now in place for independent agents and brokers. (Actual licensing could occur at either the federal or the state level.) This would ensure that all representatives understood Medicare, the products they were selling, and current restrictions on deceptive or abusive marketing practices. Of course, training and licensure would not necessarily eliminate abuses. However, they would at least ensure that representatives were not misled by their own employers as to what activities were permissible or appropriate. In addition, the option of suspending or revoking a license would give regulators an additional enforcement tool when faced with patterns of marketing abuse.

Marketing research

By collecting and reviewing plan marketing materials, HCFA is already in a position to identify any blatant attempts to discourage high-risk enrollees. However, reviewers may not be able to readily identify more subtle practices, such as targeted messages, that affect risk selection. HCFA's monitoring ability might be enhanced if it conducted market research comparable to that conducted by the plans themselves.

For example, HCFA could routinely test marketing materials, through focus groups or other means, to learn what messages are being communicated and how different types of beneficiaries—both high-risk and low-risk—respond. (It might be appropriate for HCFA to test its own information materials, as well as those developed by plans.) The feedback from such research could be used to refine HCFA's evaluation process. It might also be used to decide what types of new information would be desirable for HCFA to collect or to require of plans.

Enhanced information collection

HCFA may enhance the information it collects in a number of ways. It may collect information on the specifics of who is carrying out direct marketing (e.g., internal sales force, captive agents), how they are trained, and how they are compensated. Information could be collected on how and where plans are spending their marketing budget (types of media and the locations in which they are spending their marketing dollars). This type of information would increase HCFA's ability to identify red flags and to further refine the standards applied to participating plans.

More standardized information dissemination

While HCFA requires that plans make available certain information to beneficiaries, little is done to ensure that such information is provided in a relatively consistent and understandable format. Individual plans have little motivation to do this on their own, because their goal is to sell their health plan, not to compare it objectively to others. At the beneficiary level the result is often confusion and misunderstanding about one plan relative to another. The centerpiece of one plan's marketing message may be buried in the fine print of a coverage summary of another plan. The opportunities for misunderstandings about covered services are particularly great because Medicare allows plans to provide enhanced services and the language used to explain coverage is often highly technical. By emphasizing coverage of lower cost services and deemphasizing coverage of higher cost chronic conditions, there is tremendous opportunity to influence the risk profile of enrollees.

To at least partially address the above concerns, HCFA could be more prescriptive about how and what types of information may be presented to consumers. In the non-elderly market, groups such as health plan purchasing cooperatives (HPCs) commonly define certain categories of information that plans are required to provide in a standard format. Similar standardization requirements apply to some of the information furnished by Medigap carriers. HCFA could employ a similar approach for Medicare HMOs, requiring that coverage of certain topics in plan marketing materials conform to fixed formats.

Beneficiary surveys

Current oversight mechanisms focus on beneficiaries who *do* enroll. For example, HCFA may respond to complaints about a plan's marketing by surveying beneficiaries who have recently joined the plan or who have recently disenrolled from it. Such surveys can determine whether enrollees were inadequately informed about the consequences of enrollment. However, to uncover risk selection practices, one would need to survey beneficiaries who had some contact with the plan but *did not* enroll.

One possible—if cumbersome—way of doing so would be to require plan marketing personnel, including those responding to telephone inquiries, to maintain logs of contacts with beneficiaries. HCFA might then survey non-enrollees to learn how they made their decision and what they were told by the plan. (Of course, there would be the difficulty of ensuring that the contact logs themselves were accurate.)

Use of and Regulation of Independent Agents and Brokers[18]

Direct marketing by plans could be replaced or supplemented by marketing through intermediaries who are better able and more apt to provide objective information and marketing services across multiple health plans. Independent agents may, for example, be in a better position to play this role than salaried employees of health plans. Agents who now sell Medigap coverage might offer their clients a broader range of options, including Medicare HMOs.

However, there are several types of agents. Some are "captive agents": although not employed by the insurer, they sell exclusively for one company. Independent agents and brokers in theory do not represent the interest of any single company. In practice, however, even independent agents or brokers usually have a small group of companies with which they work predominately. Such quasi-dependence may be the result of the agent's evaluation of the health plan (its quality, service, etc.). It may be a result of the level or type of compensation provided by the plan. Some plans pay higher commissions than others. Agent commissions in the small group and individual markets range from less than 5 percent of premium to 40–50 percent of premium.[19] In many cases plans provide volume incentives and bonuses to agents. These bonuses/incentives force an independent agent to make a decision as to where he or she wants to allocate limited time and resources. The agent who offers plans across many different companies is unlikely to make a bonus quota from any of them. It is also becoming more common for health plans to require that agents write a minimum percentage of their business through the company, indirectly limiting the agent's ability to represent other plans. Finally, close ties with only a few companies are often born of necessity. Many agents and brokers find it very difficult, if not impossible, to stay abreast of all products offered by all plans. They therefore focus on a limited and manageable range of health plans and products.

If greater reliance is to be placed on agents and brokers as sources of coverage information for beneficiaries, steps may need to be taken to assure truly independent agents. HCFA might require that agents become specifically licensed to sell products to Medicare beneficiaries. Any individual selling Medicare products would have to demonstrate an ability to present all available products offered in the area in which they are issuing coverage to Medicare beneficiaries. As part of this process agents would be required to disclose, among other things, their current compensation arrangements with health plans. The education and licensing process could occur at the federal level or more locally at the state level under federal guidelines. The state approach would probably be more practical because many states already have education and licensing programs in place.

Alternatively, or additionally, HCFA could define a standard agent compensation level to ensure that agents had no incentives to steer beneficiaries to specific plans. This practice has been adopted by some of the health plan purchasing cooperatives (HPCs) now operating in the small group market. Compensation levels could be defined by HCFA directly or by relying on health plan or agent input (e.g., by averaging the compensation levels proposed or currently being used by participating health plans).

Direct Beneficiary Outreach by HCFA or Contractor

HCFA could follow the example of many state Medicaid programs by developing its own program of outreach and counseling for beneficiaries or by contracting with a third-party enrollment broker or counseling firm. Certain multi-state or national agent/broker firms could perform this function, as could state agencies—especially those that have already developed their own beneficiary counseling programs. As was noted earlier, the BBA specifically authorizes a test of this concept on a demonstration basis.

The following discussion reviews the Medicaid experience with enrollment brokers.[20] As a preliminary, however, it should be emphasized that two key differences between Medicare and Medicaid beneficiaries may limit the applicability of state experience. First, most state programs using enrollment brokers are doing so in the context of systems mandating managed care enrollment for specified groups of Medicaid beneficiaries. Beneficiaries have an incentive to seek counseling so that they can make a choice among plans, rather than be assigned arbitrarily to a plan by the state. Even so, large proportions of beneficiaries fail to make a selection. Medicare beneficiaries, who remain in the fee-for-service program by default, may be even less likely to access an enrollment broker and make decisions about coverage options.

Second, as was suggested, Medicare beneficiaries may be harder to reach. Medicaid beneficiaries must generally appear at local social services offices for periodic redetermination of benefits; this offers a logical site for enrollment choice presentations and counseling. The only comparable site for Medicare beneficiaries is Social Security offices. However, outreach at these sites would generally reach only newly eligible beneficiaries. Outreach efforts for Medicare beneficiaries would either have to rely chiefly on means other than face-to-face encounters or occur at a wide variety of sites, such as senior centers, nursing facilities, and housing developments for the elderly. This approach would be costly and would still miss many beneficiaries, such as those who are homebound.

As of January 1997, 24 of the 40 states that offer their Medicaid beneficiaries a choice of risk-reimbursed managed care plans use the services of a marketing and enrollment broker to present information about health plan choices to beneficiaries and perform the function of enrolling beneficiaries in their selected health plans. States have turned to this approach for several reasons:

- to avoid risk selection by health plans;
- to improve outreach to and education of Medicaid beneficiaries about available Medicaid coverage options;
- to curb or prevent marketing abuses by health plans that have historically occurred in Medicaid managed care programs (most states have moved or are moving to prohibit direct marketing to individual Medicaid beneficiaries by health plans and thus needed other mechanisms for outreach); and

- to achieve cost-savings (shifting this function from government employees to external contractors assisted some states in achieving downsizing and budget reduction goals).

While states report general satisfaction with their experiences with enrollment brokers, there has not been any systematic evaluation of the performance of these entities. Analysts who have studied the growth and use of enrollment brokers cite the following issues as significant:

- *Substituting sources of risk selection.* While the use of third parties may thwart attempts by health plans to select low-risk enrollees and discourage potential high users from enrolling, the use of enrollment brokers can actually assist Medicaid beneficiaries to practice their own risk selection. For example, to the extent that an enrollment broker is knowledgeable about health plan structures, special services, and care management practices, he or she may be more successful (than an individual beneficiary would be by himself or herself) at identifying for sicker individuals health plans that have stronger networks of specialty providers, hospitals, and any special care programs.

- *Role of brokers.* A consensus has not yet emerged about how enrollment brokers should communicate information on competing health plans to individual consumers. There may be agreement that brokers should not make any judgments about the relative merits of health plans or which health plan may be better for a particular beneficiary. The broker should maintain independence and objectivity, allowing individual consumers to choose based on their own decision-making processes. Yet, because there is an abundance of potential information that can be shared with individual consumers, an enrollment broker will need to make judgments about the information in which the consumer will be most interested. The very process of identifying with the consumers their individual healthcare priorities and selecting which plan information to share with consumers will require that an enrollment broker exercise judgment. Brokers will likely require extensive training and monitoring to ensure that they walk the fine line between assisting consumers to identify their own needs and priorities and providing a selective amount of information versus allowing the broker's own biases and beliefs to influence consumers' decisions.

- *Compensation of enrollment brokers.* As compensation is thought to affect delivery of healthcare, so too may it affect enrollment functions. If enrollment brokers are paid based on the number of enrollments processed in a timely manner, this can encourage quick enrollment of beneficiaries without full consideration of beneficiaries' best needs. If brokers are penalized for disenrollments (not due to loss of eligibility), brokers may be encouraged to make disenrollment more difficult for beneficiaries. (A possible solution would be to base compensation in part on consumer assessments of the brokers' performance.)

FACTORS LIMITING THE LIKELY EFFECT OF THESE OPTIONS ON RISK SELECTION

While there are in any case good reasons for curtailing marketing abuses and improving consumer information, the effects of these measures on the problem of biased selection are uncertain for several reasons.

Few measures can compare the performance of managed care plans with the performance of the fee-for-service sector. If high-risk beneficiaries are reluctant to join restrictive plans, comparison of Plan A and Plan B will do nothing to reassure them that managed care in general is not of inferior quality. Yet there may be no meaningful way of comparing managed care and fee-for-service. Any measure of quality under fee-for-service would necessarily reflect the average performance of widely varying individual providers. (This may, of course, be true in health plans as well, leading to the suggestion that comparisons would be more useful at the provider rather than the plan level. However, plans may influence performance on at least some measures.)

Comparisons of consumer satisfaction may be more feasible. Learning that enrollees in health plans are generally satisfied could be reassuring to beneficiaries who are considering enrollment for financial reasons. However, beneficiaries may understand intuitively that satisfaction, too, is largely related to the performance of individual providers. A beneficiary in the fee-for-service sector who is already personally satisfied with his or her source of care may not give much weight to aggregate figures on satisfaction in Plan A.

At the level of individual plans, fully informed choices may actually increase selection bias. If beneficiaries received sufficient information to ascertain which plan was best at treating dropsy, dropsy patients would flock to that plan.[21] This creates disincentives for superior service; unless payment is adjusted for health status a plan would do better to score as acceptable but not superior on this particular measure. It may be possible to develop more generalized measures of quality that would not invite this form of condition-specific selection. For example, blended scores might reflect plans' overall performance in broad categories of care, such as preventive services or management of chronic illness. However, it would be difficult to reach consensus on the components and weighting of such measures. Alternatively, reported measures might focus on treatment of conditions, such as heart disease or cancer, that all elderly people are concerned about whether they are immediately affected. Even so, these measures are likely to be of somewhat greater interest to beneficiaries who foresee an immediate need for care.

Measures to reduce deliberate risk selection in the enrollment process must be accompanied by measures to address induced disenrollment. Plans that cannot discourage high-risk beneficiaries from enrolling can encourage them to disenroll by limiting access to necessary services (see Chapter 8 for an extended discussion of disenrollment and risk selection). The BBA, after a phase-in period, will eliminate beneficiaries' current right to disenroll at any time; disenrollment will be allowed only during the annual open enrollment period unless the beneficiary moves out of a plan's service area or can show that the plan committed certain abuses (or under other special circumstances). Despite this change, there will remain an incentive for plans to encourage disenrollment by chronically ill beneficiaries who are likely to incur high costs over a long period. This problem can be identified relatively easily through post-disenrollment surveys, although resolving the problem is more difficult (see Chapter 8). It should also be noted that the likelihood of induced disenrollment might increase if reforms in the Medigap market were to be adopted, so that dissatisfied health plan enrollees could be assured of access to alternative coverage after disenrollment.

CONCLUSION

To advocate improved consumer information as a means of reducing selection bias assumes that higher-risk beneficiaries making fully informed and rational choices will be more likely than at present to select managed care options. This is by no means certain. Even if dissemination of information on quality created incentives for managed care plans to improve their performance, beneficiaries with sufficient means to buy conventional Medigap coverage might still rationally prefer to remain in fee-for-service. Moreover, many elderly beneficiaries might still have difficulty in understanding their options and weighing the tradeoffs involved. Over time, newly eligible Medicare beneficiaries are more likely to have had experience in choosing health plans and be better equipped to do so. For the current population, however, simple inertia and ingrained preferences are likely to mean that the phenomenon of biased selection will continue for many years.

If adequate risk adjustment mechanisms were available, biased selection might not even be a concern. So long as plans were appropriately compensated for the level of risk presented by their populations, it might be all to the good if beneficiaries selected plans that met their needs and preferences. A reliable payment system could even encourage the development of plans to meet the needs of specific populations. A fully functioning market does not necessarily produce a single, uniform product for all buyers, nor should this be expected in healthcare. In this view, the aim of information efforts would be not to eliminate selection bias but to assist consumers in making the selections that are best for them.

The new system established by the BBA makes this a more pressing concern than ever before, for several reasons. After a phase-in period, beneficiaries will have an opportunity to change their choice of plans only once a year. While this restriction will reduce opportunities for plans to encourage mid-year disenrollment by high-cost participants, it also makes it all the more important that enrollees fully understand the implications of their choice of plans at the outset.

Some of the new options expose beneficiaries to significant financial risk. MSA plans can impose a deductible of up to $6,000; there will also now be high-deductible Medigap plans. Enrollees in private fee-for-service plans could be subject to balance billing by providers, including balance billing by inpatient hospitals—never previously allowed and potentially resulting in charges of tens of thousands of dollars to some unlucky participants. It is therefore critical that beneficiaries fully understand these options.

Plans in some areas may face much greater pressure than before to cut costs. Payment for HMOs and other Medicare+Choice plans will gradually shift from area-specific rates to a national rate that will be adjusted for local input costs but not for local practice patterns. Plans operating in traditionally high-cost areas will have a very short time to achieve significant utilization reductions. Better consumer information could provide some countervailing pressure to maintain quality.

Finally, the system as a whole may be entering a period of instability. There could be significant year-to-year fluctuations in costs and benefits for specific plans, compelling beneficiaries to reevaluate their coverage choices more often. All of this will occur during a period when many beneficiaries may have a steadily shrinking disposable income available to spend on supplemental coverage.[22]

Regardless of whether or not improved payment systems are adopted, the steps that would best promote informed decision making are fairly clear:

- Neutral, third-party sources of information for beneficiaries should be developed. Of the available options, use of enrollment brokers seems preferable. If this should prove impractical for budgetary or other reasons, HCFA should encourage participation by genuinely independent agents.
- Direct marketing contact with beneficiaries by health plans should be restricted and closely monitored. In particular, means must be found

of monitoring the content of direct presentations. Targeted marketing should be limited by more careful scrutiny of plan materials and marketing strategies. Consideration should be given to regulating group presentations to unrepresentative populations. Marketing by affiliated physicians or providers should be prohibited. In the case of provider-sponsored organizations, there should at least be safeguards to prevent communication of medical information to the organization's marketing department.

- Experience with non-elderly populations suggests that informed choice is workable when the number of options is limited and standardized on key dimensions, such as benefits. If this should prove impracticable, then considerably more work will be needed to find ways of presenting multidimensional information in comprehensible formats.

- Further work on quality and satisfaction measurement must focus not simply on refining specific measures but also on developing a consensus about ways of aggregating measures to provide simple and meaningful plan comparisons. Work on comparison of the performance of the managed care and fee-for-service sectors, or of specific providers in each sector, is urgently needed.

All of these measures are feasible and are unlikely to be significantly more costly than the sizable marketing expenditures now made by plans. As was noted earlier, the BBA allows imposition of user fees on Medicare+Choice plans to pay for informational activities. If the aim is to develop a comprehensive system that provides information on all options, including Medigap and Medicare Select, assessments would be more equitably imposed on all carriers selling supplemental coverage. However, this may be politically impossible.

More broadly, adoption of any of these measures is likely to face resistance from at least some segments of the managed care industry. The industry itself must be persuaded that improving consumer choice carries some benefit. This may be most likely if health plans can be shown that current selection patterns within the managed care sector jeopardize individual plans in unpredictable ways.

Again, whether or not improved information efforts and other reform measures will affect selection bias, they deserve to be adopted on their own merits. Beneficiaries' coverage choices have an important impact on their finances and on their health. Helping them make these choices wisely should be a fundamental part of the mission of the Medicare program.

NOTES

1. The author wishes to thank his colleagues at the Institute for Health Policy Solutions for their contributions to the paper upon which this chapter is based: Ann Page, Elizabeth W. Hoy, Kevin Haugh, and Richard E. Curtis.

2. Medigap plans will not participate in the open enrollment process or pay users' fees.

3. In addition, all beneficiaries enrolled in Part B—regardless of their supplemental coverage—pay a premium of $43.80 per month in 1998.

4. The AAPCC computation includes an adjuster for Medicaid status that may be adequate to reflect changes in Medicare utilization resulting from the adoption of managed care for the Medicaid wraparound. There is no adjuster to reflect differences between beneficiaries enrolled in retiree plans and those with individual supplemental coverage.

5. About 1.3 percent of Medicare beneficiaries are currently enrolled in other forms of Medicare managed care contracts, such as cost contracts and healthcare prepayment plans. The BBA phases out these alternatives, except for employer and union plans and plans that neither provide nor arrange inpatient care.

6. The BBA also establishes "religious fraternal benefit society plans." These are not a distinct type of plan. A religious society could offer any of the Medicare+Choice models but is free to limit enrollment to its own members.

7. This was allegedly the experience under the guaranteed issue requirements imposed by the HMO Act of 1973 on federally qualified HMOs serving the nonelderly individual market. The requirements were repealed several years later precisely because HMOs complained that they could not compete with commercial carriers that were free to discriminate.

8. Section 4032 of the BBA adds, to the ten standard Medigap plans now available, two plans that may have deductibles as high as $1,500 in 1998 and 1999.

9. HCFA 1996. The plan used for comparison was Plan C, which excludes prescription drugs and preventive care. Benefits in risk HMOs vary but are generally at least comparable to Plan C.

10. For a review of available studies, see Andrews and Lake (1993).

11. Note that IPAs were treated as resembling fee-for-service because they offered broader provider choice than staff/group models. As noted above, elderly people with multiple sources of care may instead view IPAs as more closely resembling staff/group models.

12. The following discussion is largely based on HCFA's HMO/CMP Manual, Sec. 2213.

13. Independent agents also often place business with multiple insurers/plans, but unlike brokers they are generally representatives of the insurer/plan.

14. Medigap marketing rules are in section 1882 of the Social Security Act.

15. The incentives would never be as great as those faced by HMOs or other Medicare+Choice plans, because Medigap carriers can only realize profits or losses on the limited share of beneficiary costs they pay for, while profits and losses for Medicare+Choice plans are based on total beneficiary spending.

16. This section summarizes information contained in Institute of Medicine (1996) and McCormack et al. (1996).

17. Conversation with Michael Adeberg, Health Care Financing Administration.

18. See also Chapter 5 for discussion of the pros and cons and feasibility of brokers handling enrollment.

19. Plans that pay very high commissions typically do so only during the initial years. Over time commissions are graded down.
20. The following discussion is based on a personal communication from Jane Horvath, National Academy for State Health Policy, and on U.S. General Accounting Office, 1996.
21. As a practical matter, it is not clear that any of the measures yet available would allow for such an assessment. For example, a plan's rate of performance of retinal exams for diabetics is clearly not sufficient to generalize about the plan's overall quality of care for diabetics.
22. The BBA will, for example, nearly double the share of income consumed by the Part B premium by 2007 (Moon, Gage, and Evans 1997).

REFERENCES

Andrews, E., and T. Lake. 1993. *Price and Choice in the Health Care Market: A Technical Report.* Washington, DC: Mathematica Policy Research.

Feldman R., M. Finch, B. Dowd, and S. Cassou. 1989. "The Demand for Employment-Based Health Insurance Plans." *Journal of Human Resources* 24 (1): 115–42.

Frederick/Schneiders Inc. 1995. *Analysis of Focus Groups Concerning Managed Care and Medicare.* Washington, DC.

Gibbs, D. 1995. *Information Needs for Consumer Choice: Final Focus Group Report.* Charlotte, NC: Research Triangle Institute.

Health Care Financing Administration (HCFA). 1996. *Profiles of Medicare.* Baltimore.

Health Care Financing Administration (HCFA). 1997. *Medicare Managed Care National Marketing Guide.* Baltimore. Chapter IV.

Health Care Financing Administration (HCFA). 1998. *Monthly Report, Medicare Managed Care Plans.* February. www.hcfa.gov, March 1998.

Institute of Medicine. 1996. *Improving the Medicare Market—Adding Choice and Protections.* Washington, DC: National Academy Press.

Isaacs, S. L. 1996. "Consumers' Information Needs: Results of a National Survey." *Health Affairs* 15 (4): 31–41.

McCormack L., J. Schnaier, J. Lee, and S. Garfinkel. 1996. "Medicare Beneficiary Counseling Programs: What Are They and Do They Work?" *Health Care Financing Review* 18 (1): 127–40.

Mechanic D. 1989. "Consumer Choice Among Health Insurance Options." *Health Affairs* 8 (1): 138–48.

Moon, M., B. Gage, and A. Evans. 1997. *An Examination of Key Medicare Provisions in the Balanced Budget Act of 1997.* Washington, DC: Urban Institute.

National Committee for Quality Assurance. 1995. *NCQA Consumer Information Project.* Washington, DC.

National Committee for Quality Assurance. 1996. *Consumer Information Project: Medicare/Medicaid—Findings from Focus Groups.* Washington, DC.

Sofaer, S. 1995. *Issues of Concern to Medicare Beneficiaries Considering Enrollment in Managed Care Plans: A Preliminary Report on the Medicare Consumer Information Project.* Washington, DC: National Committee for Quality Assurance.

United States Congress, Office of Technology Assessment. 1988. *The Quality of Medical Care: Information for Consumers.* OTA-H-386. Washington, DC: U.S. Government Printing Office.

United States House of Representatives, Committee on Ways and Means. 1996. *Green Book: Background Material and Data on Programs within the Jurisdiction of the Committee on Ways and Means.* Washington, DC.

United States General Accounting Office (USGAO). 1996a. *Medicaid: States' Efforts to Educate and Enroll Beneficiaries in Managed Care.* GAO/HEHS-96-184. Washington, DC.

United States General Accounting Office (USGAO). 1996b. *Medigap Insurance: Alternatives for Medicare Beneficiaries to Avoid Medical Underwriting.* Letter Report, 09/10/96, GAO/HEHS-96-180. Washington, DC.

Should Medicare Managed Care Plans and Medigap Policies Have a Coordinated Open Enrollment Period?

Thomas Rice[1]

This chapter discusses the change to a coordinated open enrollment period for Medicare beneficiaries who wish to purchase Medicare managed care plans; it also discusses whether Medigap policy coverage should also be included in the open enrollment process. As part of the Balanced Budget Act (BBA) of 1997, Congress established the Medicare+Choice Program. Beginning in 1999, the program allows Medicare beneficiaries to choose among several coverage options, including health maintenance organizations (HMOs), other managed care plans, private fee-for-service plans, and medical savings accounts (MSAs). The program includes the provision of comparative information about these options to Medicare beneficiaries and the implementation of a specific coordinated open enrollment period during which they may choose to enroll in any of these choices. Medigap policies are excluded from this system of coordinated enrollment.

The BBA represents a major improvement in the Medicare enrollment process. Before this legislation, enrollment in alternatives to the traditional Medicare fee-for-service program, such as Medicare HMOs, was not coordinated. People could join at any time, but no information was readily available that allowed for the comparison of different options. Under the new coordinated open enrollment system, beneficiaries can join or switch among their Medicare+Choice plans during the open enrollment period (November of each year) without being denied coverage. Furthermore, as part of the system, critical information will be distributed to facilitate informed choices. The result is likely to be improved decision making, as beneficiaries will be able to make side-by-side comparisons of their various options.

Medigap policies, however, are not included in the new system. This chapter argues that including them as part of the coordinated open enrollment system, coupled with extensive information dissemination about both Medigap and the Medicare+Choice options, would result in beneficiaries making better choices about whether to purchase supplemental coverage. It should also lead to more people choosing managed care plans[2]—particularly HMOs—over Medigap policies, reducing the extent of favorable selection into Medicare HMOs and changing the profile of enrollees to look more like the rest of the Medicare population.

Thus, even though the Medicare+Choice program should result in significant improvements in the market, a number of problems are likely to remain, each of which is elaborated upon later in the chapter:

- *It is difficult to obtain and use information on alternative choices.* Although information about alternatives to the traditional Medicare program will now be more widely available, the same is not true of Medigap. It is relatively easy to obtain information on Medigap benefits because ten standardized benefit packages are allowed to be sold, identified with the letters A through J. However, it is not so simple to obtain premium information. About 40 states now compile a premium comparison booklet for Medigap policies. In these states beneficiaries can get the booklet from a state agency, but in most cases they are not widely distributed and many beneficiaries do not know that they are available or where to ask for them. In other states it is still necessary to contact each company individually. Even if a statewide guide is available, premium comparisons are difficult because different companies use different methods for determining future premium levels.

- *This lack of timely comparative information reduces Medicare managed care enrollment and results in favorable selection into managed care plans and a less competitive Medigap market.* If people could easily compare Medicare+Choice options with Medigap policies, one or both of two things may happen. One, more people may move from Medigap to managed care plans. Especially if high utilizers of care presently paying steep premiums for "high end" Medigap policies that cover prescription drugs switched to managed care where prescription benefits are often available at very low cost, patterns of selection could change, enabling some Medigap premiums to fall without affecting plan profitability. Direct comparisons with Medicare plans would introduce a new source of competition into the Medigap market, which could put downward pressure on Medigap premiums.

- *Many beneficiaries purchase duplicate benefits.* This has been a major problem since the enactment of Medicare. Medigap legislation approved in 1994 clarified the rules concerning sales of more than one policy to beneficiaries, effectively making it legal if certain disclosure provisions are met.

- *Those in poor health are at risk of being denied coverage or finding it unaffordable.* Because health status and income are negatively correlated, those who are in most need of supplemental protection are least likely to be able to afford it and more likely to be turned down for coverage because of preexisting health problems. This is not so much a problem with Medicare managed care plans (because they must accept nearly everyone who applies) as it is with Medigap coverage because of insurers' options to medically underwrite and experience rate premiums.

The next section provides some background on the current situation regarding Medicare supplementary policies—including the types of coverage available and their prevalence—more detail on enrollment rules for Medicare managed care plans and Medigap policies, and additional documentation of problems with the current system. The following section describes and evaluates various options for including Medigap policies as part of the coordinated open enrollment system. It also examines a number of other issues that are likely to arise in implementing coordinated open enrollment. The final section provides some overall conclusions.

THE CURRENT ENROLLMENT SYSTEM FOR MEDICARE HMOs AND MEDIGAP POLICIES

Medicare and Supplementation

The Medicare program was never designed to pay for all of the healthcare costs incurred by the elderly (and later, disabled) population. Consequently, the passage of the Medicare legislation 30 years ago brought along with it a sizeable private market to cover some of the expenses not paid for by the program.

Table 5.1 lists the gaps in Medicare coverage. Two kinds of gaps occur: covered services for which Medicare pays only a portion of the associated costs; and services that are not covered by the program. The former is composed primarily of deductibles and copayments for hospital and physician services; the two most notable examples of the latter are prescription drugs

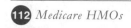

Table 5.1 Medicare Coverage Gaps

PART A

Inpatient	**1997 Payment**
Deductible for each illness spell	$760
Copayments for days 61–90	$190 per day
Copayments for lifetime reserve days 91–150	$380 per day
Beyond day 150	All costs
Skilled Nursing Facility Care	
Days 21–100	$95 per day
Beyond 100 days	All costs
Home Health Care	
Durable medical equipment	20% of approved amount
Hospice Care	
Outpatient drugs and inpatient respite care	Limited costs
Blood	
First three pints	All costs

PART B

Medical expenses	$100 annual deductible
Physician costs	20% of approved charges
Physician not accepting assignment	100% excess charges
Monthly premium	$43.80

OTHER COSTS NOT COVERED BY MEDICARE

Routine exams	All costs
Prescription drugs	
Long-term care	
Podiatric care	All costs
Care outside of the United States	All costs
All costs determined not medically necessary	All costs
Dental, hearing, and vision care	All costs

and long-term care. (Medicare does provide limited coverage for skilled nursing home care, but various restrictions are so limiting that less than 5 percent of the nursing home costs of the elderly are covered by Medicare [Public Health Service 1994].) Altogether, Medicare pays only 45 percent of the elderly population's healthcare expenditures (HCFA 1995).[3]

Consequently, the great majority of elderly Americans choose to obtain some form of supplemental healthcare coverage. A full three-quarters own some form of private coverage. Thirty-seven percent purchase this individually or through an association, 35 percent obtain it through their employer or their spouse's employer or a former employer, 7 percent have both kinds of coverage, and 12 percent have supplementation through Medicaid. Only about 11 percent of the elderly population has no form of supplementation (Chulis et al. 1993; Chulis et al. 1995).

Until recently, enrollment in Medicare HMOs was minimal. In 1985, for example, less than 4 percent of the elderly were covered by Medicare HMOs. By 1998 this figure had risen to about 14 percent and had tripled since 1992 (HCFA 1997a; HCFA 1998). In some markets, notably Riverside County and San Bernadino County in California, more than one-half of the elderly are enrolled in Medicare HMOs (HCFA 1997b). The BBA is likely to raise enrollment in managed care plans for several reasons: it expands choices beyond HMOs to preferred provider organizations as well and to a new class of health plans called provider-sponsored organizations; all Medicare beneficiaries will receive detailed information on alternative managed care choices available; and coordinating the enrollment process should lead to more competitive premiums. Finally, the legislation waives the so-called 50–50 rule, in which plans must obtain no more than 50 percent of enrollment from among Medicare and Medicaid beneficiaries. This will allow more plans to enter the market without having to be concerned about enrolling an equal number of privately insured individuals.

Historically, different types of Medicare supplemental coverage have been regulated in different ways. Medicare HMOs are licensed by states and regulated by the federal government. (The specific rules that HMOs must follow in order to comply with federal regulations are listed in Vol. 42, Part 417 of the Code of Federal Regulations.) In contrast, Medigap policies are subject to both federal and state regulation. Traditionally, state insurance departments have been responsible for regulating all insurance, including Medigap policies. There have been some instances, however, of federal intervention into the Medigap market. Most recently, under the Omnibus Budget Reconciliation Act (OBRA) of 1990, policy benefits were standardized into ten policy types (see Figure 5.1) to facilitate comparison shopping.[4] Medigap insurers are required to sell the most basic policy, Plan A, but can choose to sell any or all of the other nine policies (B–J). Policy J is the most comprehensive, covering practically all Medicare deductibles and coinsurance, as well as non-assigned services and some prescription drug costs.

Although owned by a full one-third of the elderly, the one type of supplementation that is subject to almost no regulation is supplemental coverage provided by employer group health plans. Because of the nature of employer coverage, these types of policies fall under the jurisdiction of the ERISA legislation and are therefore not subject to state regulation. Congressional legislation concerning the Medigap market does not apply to this sort of coverage. Fortunately (for their owners), these policies tend to be more comprehensive than most Medigap policies in that they are more likely to cover such things as prescription drugs,[5] mental health services, dental care, and preventive and routine services (Shea and Stewart 1995). In addition, because employers often share the cost of these policies, they tend to

Figure 5.1 Benefits Covered by Medigap Policies Under OBRA-90

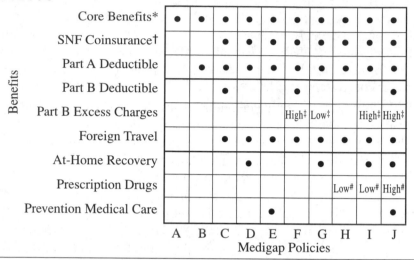

Source: NAIC, Medicare Supplement Insurance Minimum Standards Model Act (30 July 1991).

* Core benefits include coverage of all Part A (hospital) coinsurance for stays longer than 60 days, the 20 percent Part B coinsurance, and the Part A and B blood deductible.

† SNF is skilled nursing facility.

‡ Low excess charge coverage pays 80 percent of the difference between the physician's charge and the Medicare allowable rate; high coverage pays 100 percent of the difference.

Low prescription drug coverage has a $250 annual deductible, 50 percent coinsurance, and a maximum annual benefit of $1,250; high coverage is similar but it has a $3,000 maximum annual benefit.

cost the beneficiaries less than Medigap policies would. In 1992, the average annual out-of-pocket premium payment was $1,014 for Medigap policies and $728 for employer-sponsored policies (Chulis et al. 1995). However, in recent years employer subsidies have been falling: the employer share of premiums paid for retiree health insurance coverage declined by about 20 percent from 1988 to 1992 (KPMG Peat Marwick 1993).

A major concern is that employers have been pulling back on providing health insurance to retirees. In part because employers are now required to include expected liabilities of retiree health benefits in their financial statements, there has been a movement toward making these plans less costly by contributing less toward the premiums and by raising deductibles and coinsurance (Shea and Stewart 1995) or ending retiree coverage altogether. A recent survey found that the percentage of firms offering retiree health insurance coverage dropped from 40 percent in 1993 to 35 percent in 1995 (Shiels and Alecxih 1996). If employers drop coverage, former policyholders are placed in an even more difficult situation because they are likely to be well past the six-month Medigap open enrollment period. The BBA does deal with this problem to a large extent, by allowing open enrollment (within 63 days) into several of the standardized Medigap plans if an employer drops its retiree coverage.

Enrollment Rules

Medicare managed care plans

Under the BBA, nearly all individuals who are eligible for Medicare can enroll in any Medicare managed care plan that serves their geographic area, without restriction. Managed care plans may, under certain circumstances, limit their enrollment, but when they do so they are required to accept enrollees on a first-come, first-served basis until their enrollment cap is reached.

For those who join a managed care plan, the plan must provide all Medicare services in exchange for a capitation payment from HCFA, as well as the Part B premium from the beneficiary. Plans also have the option of providing additional services, and in the past most have done so; these have typically included prescription drugs, preventive care, and vision and hearing services. The plan can charge an additional premium for such services, although currently about two-thirds choose not to. The magnitude of these premiums affects how attractive the plan is compared to Medigap coverage.

As of November 1998, when coordinated open enrollment began, beneficiaries are given the opportunity to join a Medicare+Choice plan; if they do not, they will remain in the traditional Medicare fee-for-service program. Enrollment will be effective on January 1, 1999, and on January 1 of each year thereafter. The rules concerning disenrollment will change over a several year phase-in period. Until 2001, disenrollment from Medicare+ Choice plans is allowed at any time. Ultimately (after 2002), it will be allowed only during the first three months of the year, except for new eligibles and enrollees who are new to managed care, who will be able to disenroll at any time during their first year but will be subject to the same lock-in thereafter (Chapter 8 describes some other exceptions).

Medigap policies

The OBRA-90 legislation included provisions concerning the enrollment of Medicare beneficiaries into Medigap plans. It stipulated that beneficiaries would be eligible for open enrollment into any Medigap policy during their first six months of Medicare Part B eligibility. That is, during this period they are allowed to purchase any Medigap policy (plan types A–J) from any insurer without being subject to any underwriting. Consequently, they cannot be turned down for coverage during this period, and they cannot be charged more than any other person (in their age/sex rating cell). After this six-month period, insurers can evaluate health status and, as a result, deny coverage.

The BBA has several special provisions that allow beneficiaries to enroll in a Medigap policy (Plans A, B, C, or F), without restriction, after the six-month open enrollment period has elapsed. These include instances when former employers cancel their retiree insurance, when beneficiaries' Medigap insurer or health plan goes out of business, and when a person who has not been enrolled in a managed care plan before enrolls in a Medicare+Choice plan but then disenrolls within a 12-month period.

Most insurers do allow policyholders limited open enrollment when they switch from a pre-standardized (1991 or before) policy to a current policy. The General Accounting Office reports that 14 of 16 insurers that employ medical underwriting allow policyholders to switch to a standardized plan that has comparable or fewer benefits than their pre-standardized policy, without imposing any underwriting restrictions (USGAO 1996). In addition, all companies surveyed allow switching from one standardized plan type to another one with fewer benefits. If a person wishes to switch to a more comprehensive standardized plan, however, underwriting is usually employed (USGAO 1996). This enables companies to help prevent adverse selection. Regarding disenrollment, beneficiaries are given a 30-day "free look" period, during which they can return their policies for any reason and be reimbursed for their premiums.

Two other aspects of the Medigap open enrollment rules are relevant to this study. First, even though insurers cannot turn down anyone during the open enrollment period, they can impose up to a six-month preexisting condition limitation clause, in which coverage is not provided for already existing medical conditions during the first six months of policy ownership. Second, it is important to emphasize that this open enrollment period is not "coordinated" in the sense considered by this report. The open enrollment does not occur at a fixed time during the year. Instead, each person's open enrollment period consists of the first six months after they become eligible for Medicare—which, of course, would be a different set of dates for nearly everyone. Equally important, Medigap open enrollment is not annual; the open enrollment provisions are once-in-a-lifetime.

Problems with the Current System

A number of problems plague Medicare beneficiaries who are interested in obtaining supplemental coverage, four of which are discussed here.

Difficulties in obtaining and using information

The ability to make good choices hinges on the availability of reliable information about these choices. In the area of health insurance, this includes such things as the benefits covered, premiums, and the composition of the provider panel. Recently, much emphasis has also been placed on the quality of care provided and on consumer satisfaction.

Until recently, good comparative information has been difficult to obtain. Consumers typically had to obtain it from each individual company and make comparisons as best they could, and of course nothing was available on quality and satisfaction. As a result, most studies have shown low levels of beneficiary understanding of both Medicare and Medigap coverage.[6]

The exception to this was the requirement that policies be standardized into just ten different configurations. This requirement facilitated choice because different companies sell policies with identical benefits. However, it did not solve the problem entirely because information on premiums of various companies is not readily available. Even the states that compile policy comparison information that includes premiums do not distribute the information to the entire elderly population in the state. Rather, individuals must obtain the information for themselves by contacting a particular state agency.

Even if they were widely distributed, premium comparisons still would be difficult to understand because companies use different rating practices. Some use "community" rating, charging the same premium to everyone. Others use "issue-age" rating, in which the premium charged depends on the age at which people initially purchase the policy. Recently, there appears to have been an increase in a third type of rating among small and medium-sized insurers, called "attained-age." Under this method, premiums increase as the enrollee ages. Attained age rating results in less predictable future premiums as well as higher premiums when people get older and often have less income. Attained-age rating is attractive to some insurers, however, because it allows them to charge less to a 65-year-old person—increasing the chance that such a person will opt for and stay with a particular company throughout their senior years (McCormack, Fox, Rice, and Graham 1996).

Comparisons among Medicare HMOs have been even more difficult, although this should change dramatically after 1998, when the BBA requirements on information are implemented. Until now the Medicare program has not compiled HMO comparison sheets for most regions of the country. Even on the West coast, the one area in which comparative information on all Medicare HMO plan benefits and premiums has been compiled, beneficiaries have had to obtain this information from HCFA, and its existence has not been widely publicized. Current resources do not allow the agency to disseminate this information to all beneficiaries in the region.

Implementation of the BBA will change this for Medicare managed care plans country-wide. The legislation calls for the federal government to send detailed information to all Medicare beneficiaries about all Medicare+Choice plans available in their geographic area. In addition to coverage and costs, disenrollment rates and enrollee satisfaction measures are also to be included. Because enrollment will be coordinated, beneficiaries will receive information about all plan choices at one time, just before they make their enrollment decisions. Coupled with this will be a toll-free telephone number for inquiries and an Internet site. These are likely to enhance the degree to which consumers engage in comparison shopping. However, even with comparative information for all HMOs, beneficiaries may find it difficult to weigh the different benefits and costs of their options because HMO benefits are not standardized, unlike Medigap plans (see Chapter 6).

Detailed information about Medigap plans is not included in the legislation. Generally the only source of such information that is available is from state information, counseling, and assistance (ICA) programs. As part of the OBRA-90 legislation, $10 million per year is available to states to establish and/or enhance counseling activities for Medicare beneficiaries. These activities include providing assistance with completing Medicare claims and appealing coverage decisions (through telephone and in-person counseling, seminars, videos, etc.), as well as information about alternative types of Medicare supplementation, including Medigap, Medicare managed care plans, Medicaid, and long-term care insurance (McCormack, Schnaier, Lee, and Garfinkle 1996). All states receive such funding, with the amount varying by population, with an average initial award per state of $173,000 in 1992. This is very little per Medicare beneficiary—about 65 cents per person per year—although the amount spent per beneficiary actually using the service is much higher—about $46.00. (For an evaluation of the ICA programs, see McCormack et al. 1994; McCormack, Schnaier, Lee, and Garfinkle 1996.)

Beneficiaries are therefore likely to face severe obstacles in comparing their health insurance options and making informed choices. Even with detailed information, they may find it difficult to weigh and compare Medicare+Choice options. Moreover, there will still be a large information gap. They will have detailed information about their Medicare+Choice options but not about Medigap. A coordinated open enrollment period that included both sets of options would allow beneficiaries to better carry out informed comparison shopping.

Selection bias

Perhaps surprisingly, there does not appear to be adverse selection bias in the overall purchase of supplemental Medicare coverage. Most studies have found that, controlling for confounding factors such as age, sex, marital status, income, and education, beneficiaries with supplemental coverage tend to be just as healthy or healthier than those without such coverage (Cafferata 1984; Christensen, Long, and Rodgers 1987; Rice and McCall 1985; Rice, McCall, and Boismier 1991; and Taylor, Short, and Horgan 1988).[7] There may, however, be adverse selection within the Medigap market. It appears, for example, that there is adverse selection toward Medigap plans H–J, which cover prescription drugs (McCormack, Fox, Rice, and Graham 1996).

The problematic area for selection bias is between Medicare managed care plans and all other beneficiaries. Repeatedly, studies have shown that Medicare HMO enrollees tend to be healthier (as defined in a number of different ways) than other beneficiaries (Chapter 2 summarizes and cites numerous studies). This would not be such a problem if Medicare HMOs were paid on the basis of the health status of plan enrollees. But instead, payments are based on the health status of fee-for-service enrollees (Wilensky and Rossiter 1986). As a result, Medicare actually loses money on its HMO enrollees (Langwell and Hadley 1990; Brown et al. 1993). This will change to some extent with the implementation of the BBA because payment to managed care plans will be partly adjusted for risk levels of enrollees in the plan. Nevertheless, payments will still be based in part on costs in the Medicare fee-for-service program (Chapter 3 provides more details).

A coordinated open enrollment system is likely to decrease selection bias, particularly among people who do not own supplementary coverage. Currently, Medicare beneficiaries without any private insurance coverage (employer-based, Medigap, or Medicare HMO) tend to have lower incomes, be non-white, report poorer health status, and have more functional limitations (Chulis, Eppig, and Poisal 1995). Although many have attachments to their physicians, they also are likely to find their current out-of-pocket costs to be quite burdensome. By providing information on the availability of Medicare managed care plans in their area—most of which require no premium payments beyond the Medicare Part B premium and have minimal copayments for services—more of these people are likely to join, thus reducing the amount of favorable selection.

To the extent that a coordinated open enrollment system increases Medicare managed care enrollment generally, it may reduce the extent of favorable selection into plans. This is because the pool of beneficiaries who have not yet joined tend to be less healthy. Currently, beneficiaries with significant health problems are disproportionately in the fee-for-service system. Providing timely, comparable information on cost and quality is likely to encourage more beneficiaries to join managed care plans. As HMO membership grows it may more closely resemble the Medicare population as a whole. However, because a small number of people account for a large volume of all expenditures, as discussed in Chapter 2, considerable favorable selection can occur even with high HMO penetration rates.

Purchase of duplicate benefits

Since the beginning of Medicare, duplicate supplemental coverage has been a problem. It is estimated that in 1991, about 3 million beneficiaries paid $1.8 billion for duplicate coverage (USGAO 1994). There are several possible reasons for this:

- Many beneficiaries have coverage through their employer and do not understand that they do not require additional coverage.
- The confusing nature of Medicare and Medigap benefits makes it difficult for beneficiaries to understand what constitutes adequate coverage.
- Although various disclosure requirements now must be met before an agent or company can sell a Medigap policy to seniors who already have coverage, it continues to be legal to sell duplicative policies to beneficiaries. As a result, many people buy duplicative coverage.

Although a beneficiary could not by law be covered by more than one Medicare HMO at a time, it is quite possible that he or she could own a Medigap policy in addition to HMO coverage. Unfortunately, few data are available on the extent of this problem. Enactment of a coordinated open enrollment system could reduce the extent of duplicate coverage because all new policy purchases would happen during the same period. This may make it easier for beneficiaries to decide whether a particular policy purchase is indeed necessary.

Denial of coverage

One problem faced by Medicare beneficiaries concerns their inability to change plans. As noted earlier, the vast majority of Medigap insurers allow policyholders to switch to a less comprehensive policy without imposing any underwriting limitations. However, 11 of 25 of the largest Medigap insurers surveyed in 1996 used medical underwriting for beneficiaries who apply for coverage after the six-month open enrollment period, and five more used it for some policies (such as those covering prescription drugs) (USGAO 1996). Only nine guaranteed enrollment for all of their policies. In general, Blue Cross and Blue Shield plans provided guaranteed enrollment, while commercial insurers did not.

Until passage of the BBA, if a person wished to leave a Medicare managed care plan, or if his or her retiree coverage was terminated, there was no guarantee of obtaining Medigap after the six-month open enrollment period had elapsed. The BBA allows beneficiaries to purchase a Medigap policy within 63 days of losing their retiree benefits or of terminating their enrollment in a Medicare+Choice plan so long as they were in that plan for no longer than a year. This should encourage some beneficiaries with serious health problems to try a Medicare+Choice plan by providing reassurance that they will be able to regain Medigap coverage if the HMO turns out to be unsatisfactory.

COORDINATED OPEN ENROLLMENT SHOULD INCLUDE MANAGED CARE PLANS AND MEDIGAP POLICIES

Description of Proposal

This section describes and evaluates a number of options for a coordinated open enrollment period for Medicare beneficiaries that would encompass Medigap policies as well as Medicare managed care plans. The Medicare+Choice provisions of the BBA are taken as a given, and our proposal is to broaden the system to include Medigap policies in the coordinated open enrollment period.

In summary, we propose that during November of each year all Medicare managed care plans and Medigap policies be required to conduct a one-month open enrollment period. Prior to November, information would be distributed to all Medicare beneficiaries about the upcoming open enrollment period. This would include details on the HMO and Medigap options available to people in their geographic area, who to contact for more information, and how to enroll. In addition, various forums would be held in the months prior to November where beneficiaries could hear more about their options and could ask questions. A toll-free number would provide the same service continuously for several months prior to November.

During November, actual enrollment would occur. Whether directly with the insurer or HMO or through a designated broker that contracts with Medicare (discussed below), beneficiaries could sign up for a health plan without any restrictions. Those not choosing a plan would remain in the traditional Medicare fee-for-service program. They would remain without supplementation unless they already had supplemental coverage from an employer or former employer.

Direct Enrollment versus Use of Third-Party Broker

One of the key decisions in implementing a coordinated open enrollment system is the extent to which third-party brokers (under contract with Medicare) should be involved in the process.[8] We evaluate coordinated enrollment of both Medigap and managed care with a broker handling enrollment, as well as the more limited possibility of using a broker only for enrolling people in Medicare managed care plans and Medigap coverage still being purchased directly through the company.

There are three main activities that brokers could carry out: disseminating information, answering queries, and carrying out the enrollment process. We focus on the last of these activities because it is the most crucial.

The BBA is very cautious in this area and only calls for HCFA to conduct a demonstration project that would include examination of a brokering process. The reason for such a limited step was probably because this is highly contentious, in part because it is in sharp contrast with the status quo. Currently, people sign up with Medicare managed care plans and Medigap companies directly. In the case of Medicare HMOs, the HMO informs HCFA so that the details of the risk contract and the capitated payment can be arranged. For Medigap policies, the company does not have to inform HCFA (although it does provide annual summary statistics to the National Association of Insurance Commissioners as well as to state insurance departments).

If brokers were used to conduct enrollment, beneficiaries would contact the broker and state their enrollment decision. They would then be sent a more detailed enrollment form to complete, which, among other things, would indicate the rules they would have to follow, as well as their agreement to keep up with premium payments. Then the broker would inform the company, which would contact the enrollee to provide a copy of the insurance contract and/or other materials, make any additional arrangements for receiving premium payment, and perhaps arrange for an initial need-assessment screening examination.

EVALUATION OF ALTERNATIVES

Coordinated Open Enrollment for Medicare Managed Care Plans and Medigap Policies

This subsection will evaluate the advantages and disadvantages of a coordinated open enrollment system for Medicare managed care plans and Medigap policies together in comparison to the status quo—that is, the system enacted by the BBA in which there is coordinated open enrollment for Medicare+Choice plans only.

The overriding benefit of such a system is that it would provide consumers with much better, complete information about alternative health insurance choices. As noted throughout this chapter, under the current system it is difficult for Medicare beneficiaries to engage in effective comparison shopping. Medicare HMOs and Medigap policies offer very different sorts of benefits, require different premiums (often using different premium rating practices), and conduct marketing activities at different times. Furthermore, there is no centralized national telephone number to obtain the information needed to make valid comparisons across Medicare managed care and Medigap policies. Beneficiaries are forced to contact each company separately or seek the help of ICA programs, which have only had funding to provide this information to a small percentage of program beneficiaries.

This is in stark contrast to the information that could be made available under a coordinated open enrollment system. During November, every Medicare beneficiary would be sent information that compared the benefits, premiums, and other policy features not only of all competing Medicare managed care plans but also of all Medigap policies in their areas. They would be notified of a toll-free number that they could call to ask any questions. Although the success of such a system cannot be ascertained before the fact, it is likely that it would dramatically improve beneficiaries' knowledge of the relative advantages of managed care versus Medigap and thus promote better health insurance choices.

The quality of information could be improved under this system. Currently, much if not most information about health insurance choices is obtained from the companies themselves or their representatives. The BBA calls for objective comparative information for managed care plans, but there is no good source for Medigap policies. By involving an objective source of information—the Medicare program or its designated broker—one would expect that the information provided would be less biased. This is particularly true of verbal information, which can easily be presented selectively or even distorted by insurers and their agents.

A second advantage is that it would likely increase the number of beneficiaries with access to Medicare managed care coverage. By giving consumers information on the benefits and costs of managed care compared to Medigap policies, more will consider managed care coverage, which provides more comprehensive benefits and could cost $1,000 or even $2,000 less per year than comparable Medigap coverage.[9] In essence, the managed care plans are getting free advertising disseminated to all beneficiaries through the provisions of the BBA, although the information does not promote any particular plan. Under the proposal described here, beneficiaries would see their Medigap benefits compared to the managed care options. To the extent that this stimulates more beneficiaries to switch from Medigap to managed care, it could encourage more managed care plans to enter the marketplace.[10]

Medigap companies would face additional competitive pressure if managed care options were clearly brought to the attention of all beneficiaries. Because managed care plans tend to offer benefits in addition to the basic

Medicare package, often without extra cost beyond the Part B premium, Medigap insurers would face pressure to lower their premiums or face losing market share.

A third advantage of a coordinated open enrollment system is that it would likely reduce the amount of favorable selection experienced by Medicare managed care plans in general and HMOs in particular. To the extent that coordinated open enrollment increases beneficiary awareness of the potential savings of HMOs compared to Medigap coverage, more people will consider choosing HMOs instead of Medigap policies. In addition, showcasing HMOs' benefits (and their low costs) to those without any supplemental coverage should pique their interest. Because Medigap enrollees and those who currently have no supplemental coverage tend to be less healthy than those in Medicare HMOs, an increase in the popularity of HMOs should result in the HMO population more closely reflecting the health status of the overall elderly population—that is, in less favorable selection. (However, as noted earlier and in Chapter 2, selection bias could well persist even with much higher HMO market penetration.)

A fourth advantage is that fewer beneficiaries are likely to purchase duplicate coverage. If all purchases are made at the same time each year, beneficiaries may realize that purchasing one policy at a time is enough.

A fifth advantage of coordinated open enrollment is that it would improve access to care for those in poor health. Although Medigap policies are now required to offer open enrollment during the first six months of Part B enrollment, beneficiaries still face significant underwriting restrictions. Most importantly, if they do not purchase a policy during this six-month window, they are not guaranteed open enrollment ever again in the Medigap market. With coordinated open enrollment, individuals could purchase a Medigap policy in any given year, during open enrollment. In addition, the BBA allows people wishing to switch back to Medigap policies to do so (within 12 months) if they find themselves dissatisfied with their managed care plans. That should also encourage managed care enrollment because beneficiaries face less risk in giving managed care a try, knowing that they can regain their original Medigap policies.

There are some disadvantages to coordinated open enrollment, however. First, some beneficiaries may be overwhelmed by the volume of information on alternative health plans that they receive; this could result in poor choices or in inducing excessive worry about health insurance choices. Another problem does not concern the system itself, but it is the likely political reaction to bringing Medigap into the same enrollment system. Medigap insurers are likely to oppose it because: (a) it could well reduce their market share as more beneficiaries join managed care plans; (b) it may result in lower profit, not only because of additional competition, but also because more beneficiaries will become aware of premium differences among different Medigap companies; (c) they do not want older and sicker beneficiaries to have the privilege of guaranteed enrollment on an annual basis; and (d) they do not want more federal government involvement in the market. One would anticipate especially strong opposition from insurance agents, as this would result in a considerable diminution of their roles.

Other Issues

Direct enrollment versus third-party broker

The issue being considered here is whether a third-party broker should be used to actually conduct enrollment. That is, if a person wishes to enroll in a Medicare+Choice plan or buy a Medigap policy, he or she would contact the broker to enroll. The broker would in turn pass this information on to the managed care plan or Medigap company and, in the case of managed care enrollment, to HCFA.

The use of a broker for enrollment is a politically sensitive issue because it puts government directly in between the health plan/insurer and the beneficiary. In the case of Medigap insurance, it is totally unnecessary for sign-up to occur through a broker. The purchase of a Medigap policy has almost no direct effect on the Medicare program; there are few reasons for involving government in the enrollment process. One possible reason—to remove contact between companies/agents and prospective buyers—would probably do little to reduce misinformation or sales pressure, unless government were to take an even bigger, and more unlikely, step—banning the marketing of Medigap insurance.

The case of broker involvement in managed care enrollment is more complicated. There is no direct evidence that the current system—in which beneficiaries enroll directly with their Medicare managed care plans—does not work. But there is one major concern: the potential for plans to sign up healthy beneficiaries and avoid sick, high-risk ones. Beneficiaries who have to enroll directly through the health plan may be subject to high-pressure sales pitches or may be subtly screened and discouraged from joining. If enrollment is done through a broker, this would be less of a concern.

Managed care plans are likely to react quite negatively, however, to the prospect of being unable to enroll their beneficiaries—opposition that could make it difficult for the coordinated open enrollment proposal to be enacted. Furthermore, a demonstration project that HCFA conducted between 1985 and 1988 in Portland, Oregon, in which Medicare HMO enrollment and marketing were handled by a broker, did not appear to reduce selection bias (Porell and Turner 1990). Consequently, weighing all the factors, it would be best to conduct Medicare+Choice enrollment through two channels: directly with the plan, and through a broker, leaving the choice to the beneficiaries. Furthermore, to reduce the chance that plans try to filter out sicker beneficiaries, they should continue to be prohibited from asking any questions about beneficiary health status when carrying out the enrollment process. The threat of large fines and possible loss of their risk contracts may help deter such screening. Conclusions about the use of brokers are tentative, however, because future HCFA demonstration projects should shed additional light on this important issue.

Premium rate increases

Premium rates are set by insurers in three ways (described earlier): community rating, issue-age rating, and attained-age rating. Under the first of these, everyone is charged the same premium; under the second, everyone who purchases the policy at a particular age is charged the same amount; and under the third, people are charged more as they age. Medicare managed care plans are required to employ community rating, but Medigap insurers can use any method they wish except in a handful of states that have banned the attained-age or issue-age rating. Recent evidence from the Medigap market indicates an increase in attained-age rating among small and medium-sized carriers over the past few years because insurers are able to charge a lower premium at age 65, which may appear enticing (McCormack, Fox, Rice, and Graham 1996). Regulators tend to dislike this practice because it means that premiums will rise when the beneficiary ages, which often coincides with a period of lower disposable income. In addition, when different companies use different rating practices, consumers have difficulty comparing the benefits and costs of alternative policies.

To enable apples-to-apples comparisons among Medicare managed care plans and Medigap policies, as well as to put them on a level playing field, it is necessary that each have the same age rating requirements. This would entail either liberalizing rules for the managed care plans or making them stricter for Medigap policies. Both community rating and issue-age rating are reasonable practices (although issue-age rating is likely to inhibit beneficiaries from changing plans as they age). For the reasons noted above, it would not seem wise to allow attained-age rating to continue in the Medigap market or to be used in Medicare managed care plans.

Whether community or attained-age rating should be adopted is really a philosophical question. Under attained-age rating, people pay an amount equal to the actuarial risk associated with people their own age. Under community rating, younger people tend to subsidize older ones because the same premium is charged but the latter group tends to use more (and most costly) services. Some may view this as unfair and, furthermore, as resulting in a less than optimal amount of insurance purchasing among the younger group. However, because younger elderly people may be better able to afford coverage, it could be argued that this sort of cross-subsidy is desirable from a policy standpoint. Nevertheless, whichever method is chosen, it should apply to both Medicare managed care plans and Medigap policies (assuming, of course, that both are part of the coordinated open enrollment system).

Making managed care plans and Medigap premium rating practices comparable could have an effect on the extent of selection bias into HMOs, however. Under community (and to some extent, issue-age) rating, older beneficiaries are essentially being subsidized by younger ones. This is already happening in Medicare HMOs. But by putting Medigap policies on the same system, younger beneficiaries who have been paying lower, attained-age premiums will see a substantial rise in the cost of their Medigap policies. This could encourage some of them to join HMOs (whose premiums may now seem more attractive), reinforcing favorable selection.

Necessary resources

No attempt is made here to thoroughly examine the issue of resources necessary for the proposed implementation of coordinated open enrollment. Just a few general issues are touched upon.

Very few additional public resources should be necessary to implement the incremental proposals in this chapter because the BBA already requires that all beneficiaries be sent detailed information about the Medicare+Choice plans in their areas. The primary additional cost to the government of implementing the program proposed here is the inclusion of materials on the Medigap policies offered in each geographic area. Because companies already report this information annually to the National Association of Insurance Commissioners, additional costs (outside of preparing and mailing a heavier package) should be negligible. Another cost would be additional training to staff at the toll-free number, who would need to be familiar with Medigap as well as managed care plans.

It is difficult to estimate how costs may change for managed care plans and Medigap insurers. On the one hand, they may be reduced because marketing would be focused on a single period of the year, and much of the necessary factual information would already be distributed by Medicare or its broker. In addition, because open enrollment means no underwriting, those costs would be greatly reduced. However, depending on how the attractiveness of each changed and induced a change in enrollment and in the risk profile of enrollees in each plan, there would be adjustment and turnover costs and an impact on profitability.

CONCLUSIONS

This chapter has argued that instituting a joint coordinated open enrollment system for Medicare HMOs and Medigap policies is likely to result in a number of major improvements in healthcare coverage for the elderly. These include a wider choice of plans, the availability of more coverage options to those in poor health especially, better information, improved decision making, less selection bias, less purchase of duplicative coverage, and lower premiums through enhanced price competition. Few disadvantages weigh against these gains.

Regarding the enrollment process, the use of a broker is not necessary for Medigap policies. However, brokers should be employed in the Medicare managed care plan enrollment process, although it is pragmatically recommended that plans continue to be allowed to sign up members as well.

We expect that the coordinated open enrollment system proposed here is likely to reduce favorable selection bias in HMOs. It was concluded that, by showcasing the extensive benefits and low costs of HMOs and other managed care plans and juxtaposing them with Medigap policies premiums and benefits, coordinated open enrollment will result in many beneficiaries, who previously either owned Medigap policies or did not own any supplemental coverage, choosing HMOs or other managed care plans. Because both groups tend, on average, to be in poorer health than current HMO enrollees, their movement into HMOs will reduce the amount of favorable selection bias. Two aspects of the proposal could, however, result in more favorable selection into managed care plans. First, requiring Medigap policies to accept all applicants could result in greater adverse selection into the Medigap market. Because most beneficiaries with heavy needs already have Medigap coverage, however, it is not obvious that this would be a major problem. In addition, by giving beneficiaries the assurance that they can re-enroll in their Medigap policy if they are unhappy about their managed care plan, less favorable selection into HMOs may result. Second, by requiring Medigap policies and managed care plans to use the same premium rating system, younger beneficiaries who currently enjoy low attained-age ratings for their Medigap policies would no longer find such policies to be such a bargain and may switch to managed care.

In summary, one of the most important choices a Medicare beneficiary must make is what type (if any) of supplemental coverage to purchase. The current system is severely flawed because it is so difficult for beneficiaries to make effective decisions about which option is best. By instituting a coordinated open enrollment system for Medicare HMOs and Medigap policies, the federal government could vastly improve the quality of beneficiary choices.

NOTES

1. The research presented in this chapter was supported by the Commonwealth Fund. I would like to thank Richard Kronick, Joy de Beyer, Lauren

McCormack, and Leslie Greenwald for their helpful comments. All conclusions, however, are my own and do not reflect those of these reviewers or of the Commonwealth Fund.

2. Throughout the chapter, we refer to the Medicare+Choice options as "managed care plans." This is not strictly true because two of the options—private fee-for-service plans and MSAs—are based on fee-for-service. It is unlikely, however, that either of these options will be chosen by many beneficiaries. Very few have thus far chosen MSAs, probably because of their high deductibles, and private fee-for-service plans are unlikely to be attractive because physicians will be able to charge far more than they currently do. However, in rural areas affected by the $367 per month payment floor, private fee-for-service plans may well be attractive. Even so, relatively small numbers of beneficiaries will be involved.

3. This includes the costs of long-term care. The percentage is considerably higher if long-term care costs are excluded.

4. For more information on this legislation see Fox, Rice, and Alecxih (1995).

5. For example, whereas less than 20 percent of Medigap policies cover prescription drugs, more than 90 percent of employer-based retirement polices do (Long 1994).

6. There is a limited amount of research on how much elderly beneficiaries know about their Medigap policies; even less is known about knowledge of Medicare HMOs. Although this literature is somewhat dated, the Medigap studies show low levels of understanding of both Medicare and supplemental health insurance benefits (Cafferata 1984; McCall, Rice, and Sangl 1986).

7. This does *not* imply the absence of moral hazard; strong evidence indicates that ownership of supplemental insurance increases service usage (Christensen, Long, and Rodgers 1987; Taylor, Short, and Horgan 1988; McCall et al. 1991).

8. There would not have to be just one broker for the entire country. Medicare could contract with a different broker in different regions of the country—which may be advantageous not only to encourage competition among brokers but also because some organizations are more familiar with different local areas.

9. In California, most of the Medicare HMOs charge no premium in the large urban areas. In counties where HMOs charge premiums, these averaged around $240 per year in 1997. Most include prescription drug benefits. If purchased through the AARP in 1998, Medigap Plan H, which provides comparable benefits to many HMO plans, cost $2,016 per year in San Diego and $1,512 in the bay area. Medigap Plan J cost $2,385 in San Diego and $1,788 in San Francisco.

10. Changes in rules, notably elimination of the 50–50 rule mentioned earlier, will also encourage more managed care plans to participate in Medicare, particularly in areas with zero or very low Medicare managed care penetration.

REFERENCES

Brown, R. S., D. G. Clement, J. W. Hill, S. M. Retchin, and J. W. Bergeron. 1993. "Do Health Maintenance Organizations Work for Medicare?" *Health Care Financing Review* 15 (1): 7–23.

Cafferata, G. L. 1984. "Knowledge of Their Health Insurance Coverage by the Elderly." *Medical Care* 22 (9): 835–47.

Christensen, S., S. H. Long, and J. Rodgers. 1987. "Acute Health Care Costs for the Aged Medicare Population: Overview and Policy Options." *Milbank Quarterly* 65 (3): 397–425.

Chulis, G. S., F. J. Epping, M. O. Hogan, D. R. Waldo, and R. H. Arnett III. 1993. "Health Insurance and the Elderly: Data from the MCBS." *Health Care Financing Review* 14 (3): 163–81.

Chulis, G. S., F. J. Eppig, and J. A. Poisal. 1995. "Ownership and Average Premiums for Medicare Supplemental Insurance Policies." *Health Care Financing Review* 17 (2): 255–75.

Fox, P. D., T. Rice, and L. Alecxih. 1995. "Medigap Regulation: Lessons for Health Care Reform." *Journal of Health Politics, Policy, and Law* 20 (1): 31–48.

Health Care Financing Administration (HCFA). 1995. "Medicare—A Profile." Washington, DC.

Health Care Financing Administration (HCFA). 1997a. "Managed Care in Medicare and Medicaid." Fact Sheet. http://www.hcfa.gov/facts/f960900.htm. March 1998.

Health Care Financing Administration (HCFA). 1997b. "Market Penetration Survey—September 1997." Washington, DC.

Health Care Financing Administration (HCFA). 1998. "Medicare Managed Care Monthly Report, February 1998." http://www.hcfa.gov/stats/monthly.htm. March 1998.

KPMG Peat Marwick. 1993. *Retiree Health Benefits: An Era of Uncertainty.* Washington, DC.

Langwell, K. M., and J. P. Hadley. 1990. "Insights from the Medicare HMO Demonstrations." *Health Affairs* 9 (1): 74–84.

Long, S. H. 1994. *Prescription Drug Coverage and the Elderly: Issues and Options.* Washington, DC: American Association of Retired Persons, Public Policy Institute.

McCall, N., T. Rice, and J. Sangl. 1986. "Consumer Knowledge of Medicare and Supplemental Health Insurance Benefits." *Health Services Research* 20 (6): 633–57.

McCall, N., T. Rice, J. Boismer, and R.West. 1991. "Private Health Insurance and Medical Care Utilization: Evidence from the Medicare Population." *Inquiry* 28 (3): 276–87.

McCormack, L. A., J. A. Schnaier, A. J. Lee, S. A. Garfinkel, and M. Beaven. 1994. *Information, Counseling and Assistance Programs.* Final report submitted to the Office of Beneficiary Services, Health Care Financing Administration. Waltham, MA: Health Economics Research, Inc.

McCormack, L. A., P. D. Fox, T. Rice, and M. L.Graham. 1996a. "The Medigap Reform Legislation of 1990: Have the Objectives Been Met?" *Health Care Financing Review* 18 (1): 157–74.

McCormack, L. A., J. A. Schnaier, A. J. Lee, and S. A. Garfinkle. 1996b. "Medicare Beneficiary Counseling Programs: What Are They and Do They Work?" *Health Care Financing Review* 18 (1): 127–40.

Porell, F. W., and W. M. Turner. 1990. "Biased Selection under an Experimental Enrollment and Marketing Medicare HMO Broker." *Medical Care* 28 (7): 604–15.

Public Health Service, U.S. Department of Health and Human Services. 1994. *Health United States, 1993.* Hyattsville, MD.

Rice, T., and N. McCall. 1985. "The Extent of Ownership and the Characteristics of Medicare Supplemental Policies." *Inquiry* 22 (2): 188–200.

Rice, T., N. McCall, and J. M. Boismier. 1991. "The Effectiveness of Consumer Choice in the Medicare Supplemental Insurance Market." *Health Services Research* 26 (2): 223–46.

Shea, D. G., and R. P. Stewart. 1995. "Demand for Insurance by Elderly Persons: Private Purchases and Employer Provision." *Health Economics* 4 (4): 315–26.

Shiels, J., and L. Alecxih. 1996. *Recent Trends in Employer Health Insurance Coverage and Benefits.* Prepared for the American Hospital Association, Chicago, IL.

Taylor, A. K., P. F. Short, and C. M. Horgan. 1988. "Medigap Insurance: Friend or Foe in Reducing Medicare Deficits." In *Health Care in America,* edited by H. E. Frech III. San Francisco: Pacific Research Institute for Public Policy.

United States General Accounting Office (USGAO). 1994. *Health Insurance for the Elderly: Owning Duplicate Policies Is Costly and Unnecessary.* GAO/HEHS-94-185. Washington, DC.

United States General Accounting Office (USGAO). 1996. *Medigap Insurance: Alternatives for Medicare Beneficiaries to Avoid Medical Underwriting.* GAO/HEHS-96-180. Washington, DC.

Wilensky, G. R., and L. F. Rossiter. 1986. "Patient Self-Selection in HMOs." *Health Affairs* 5 (1): 66–80.

6

Benefit Diversity in Medicare: Choice, Competition, and Selection

Mark McClellan and Sontine Kalba[1]

Q uestions about benefit diversity in Medicare have received less attention in recent policy discussions than have other pressing issues for Medicare reform. Yet determining the content and diversity of health plans from which beneficiaries may choose is among the most challenging issues facing benefit managers for large employers and other purchasing groups. The system of health plan choice that a purchaser adopts can have major implications for health plan competition, risk selection, and the well-being of different kinds of beneficiaries, in both private plans and Medicare.

Many private healthcare purchasers have restricted the diversity of health plans offered. Such restrictions on diversity are a common feature of "managed competition" reforms (Enthoven 1993). Benefit standardization has two principal benefits. First, it promotes competition among plans. Because the various available plans provide benefits that are nominally identical, potential enrollees do not have to worry so much about reading the "fine print" of an insurance contract to make sure the benefits they actually receive turn out as expected. Many features of a health plan—such as provider availability and financial incentives, the size of plan networks, and a range of other dimensions of quality—are difficult to standardize completely. But standardization of the basic features of a health plan reduces the dimensions in which plans can vary, making it easier for potential enrollees to shop around. Second, standardization reduces the problem of risk selection.[2] With identical benefits or only a limited set of benefit options, plans have fewer opportunities to offer benefits that are more or less valued by different kinds of enrollees, to attract enrollees that are likely to use less medical care.

Benefit standardization also has costs. While enrollees in standardized systems may have a considerable range of choices among health plans, their ability to choose different levels or kinds of health insurance coverage is sharply limited. Such diversity of health insurance plan options may be valuable for the same reason that different individuals prefer different kinds of cars or other employee benefits, such as pensions. People have different tastes for health insurance. To the extent that tastes for health and healthcare vary, standardized benefits may make beneficiaries worse off.

This chapter considers the tradeoffs in choice and diversity of health plans. In the next section, we review the advantages of and obstacles to choice and diversity of health plan benefits, including some recent private-sector reform experiences. This provides a framework for our review of the current status of benefit diversity in Medicare, including Medicare's experiences with limiting diversity in the Medigap market and with promoting competition among plans that offer different benefits. We then consider some key issues for reforming Medicare plan choice and plan diversity and their likely consequences for risk selection and Medicare costs.

DIVERSITY OF BENEFITS: THEORETICAL AND PRACTICAL ISSUES

Dimensions of Diversity and Standardization

Medical services are very complex and diverse, and as a result health plans can differ in an enormous number of dimensions. Table 6.1 describes some of them. This may create considerable confusion and time costs for beneficiaries who are choosing among plans. Lowering the costs of comparing plans is a principal motivation for standardizing benefits by specifying common coverage requirements for alternative plans.

These dimensions of health plan benefits differ in ease of standardization, that is, in the extent to which an insurance purchaser can effectively mandate that health plans provide identical coverage for the benefit. Ease of standardization is largely a function of the information required for effective regulation; more complex information implies more difficulty in regulation. For example, it is relatively easy to standardize the copayments and deductibles that a plan may charge; an insurance purchaser or benefi-

Table 6.1 Some Dimensions of Health Plan Benefits

Plan Benefit Dimension	Ease of Standardization
Out-of-pocket payments (copayments, deductibles, maximum limits)	Easy
Prescription coverage	Intermediate
Well care and preventive coverage	Intermediate
Mental health coverage	Intermediate
Rehabilitation coverage	Intermediate
Nursing home coverage	Intermediate
Coverage of new or "experimental" technologies	Intermediate
Out-of-network coverage	Intermediate
Provider payment incentives	Hard
Provider utilization review	Hard
Size and quality of provider networks	Hard
Standards of care for treatment of particular diseases	Hard

ciary can easily verify the copayments or deductibles for particular services. In contrast, even if a plan is required to provide certain types of inpatient or outpatient mental health coverage, the plan may implement preadmission requirements, selective provider contracts, and other forms of utilization review that effectively limit the availability and generosity of its mental health benefits for different types of enrollees. Similarly, a plan may nominally provide prescription drug benefits, but differences across plans in participating pharmacies and formularies may result in substantial differences in the actual value of two drug benefits that appear identical. Many incentives affecting healthcare providers in a plan are complex. These include provider payment incentives (e.g., features of provider contracts such as capitation rates or supplemental payments for various services) and nonfinancial burdens on providers (e.g., the strictness of pre-certification or utilization review programs). The size and quality of the provider networks in a plan may also vary considerably. No simple rules exist for standardizing any of these dimensions of managed care benefits.

The difficulty in standardizing these benefits reflects the fact that, though all plans are required to cover "medically necessary" care, definitions of "medically necessary" differ in practice. As a result, plans that appear identical in dimensions that are relatively easy to standardize may actually provide different benefits. These hard-to-standardize features such as extent of physician choice and physician control over treatment and referral decisions are highly valued by many enrollees (Chakraborty, Ettenson, and Gaeth 1994).

Despite the obstacles, many insurance purchasing groups have successfully standardized numerous dimensions of health plans. Experience with benefit standardization in both the private sector and in markets for Medicare supplemental insurance suggests that standardization may substantially increase the responsiveness of individuals' health plan choices to the benefits and prices offered by alternative plans, thereby improving competition among plans. Before turning to that evidence, however, we consider some problems associated with benefit standardization.

Costs of Limiting Benefit Diversity: Differences in Preference

The costs of restrictions on benefit diversity depend on the extent to which the restrictions prohibit plan choices that otherwise would have been available and would have been preferred by some beneficiaries. Just as tastes differ for many other goods and services, individuals value various health benefits differently. We review three sources of differences in preferences for health plan benefits: differences arising from different expectations about use of healthcare during the coming enrollment period, differences arising from variations in income and socioeconomic status, and differences in tastes unrelated to these factors.

Individuals with the same income and health status may have different preferences about health plan benefits for many reasons. There is some evidence from economic studies that risk aversion—that is, the extent to which individuals prefer more certainty about their out-of-pocket expenditures on healthcare and other goods to less—varies considerably (Litzenberger and Ronn 1986; Szpiro 1986). Individuals who are more risk averse will prefer more generous insurance benefits. There is less evidence on the extent to which preferences about the availability of particular types of medical services such as mental health benefits, organ transplantation, or home health benefits differ across individuals in similar health.[3] Preferences may differ for many reasons, including differences in tastes for intensive medical interventions versus alternative approaches to dealing with illness, the availability of alternatives such as family members and friends to supportive medical services like home health and rehabilitation benefits, different likelihood of travel (and therefore different needs for out-of-area coverage), and different degrees of geographical access to various types of medical providers. Developing more evidence on these differences in preferences would be a useful area for further research.

Large as these differences in preferences may be, however, they are likely to be overshadowed by even greater differences in preferences about insurance benefits resulting from differences in socioeconomic status and health. For example, Garber and Phelps (1997) estimate that the optimal cost-effectiveness ratio for deciding whether a medical intervention is worthwhile is approximately 75 percent higher for an individual with annual income of $29,000 compared to an individual with annual income of $18,000. Thus, individuals with higher incomes are likely to prefer insurance benefits that imply a more generous notion of "medically necessary" care.[4]

Even more importantly, individuals who expect to have high medical expenditures while they are enrolled in a plan will strongly prefer health insurance plans that provide the most generous coverage of treatments for their disease. Individual differences that persist from one year to the next explain more than 20 percent of the variation in Medicare expenditures in any given year (Newhouse et al. 1989), so that heavy use of medical care in one year implies heavy use of medical care in the next. In addition, elective expenditures that may be deferred—such as joint replacement (and the associated rehabilitation costs) or vision care—are also an important component of Medicare expenditures. Considerable evidence from both the elderly and non-elderly suggests that chronic illnesses and expectations about use of elective services are major determinants of health plan choices, leading to differences in health risks across plans that differ in benefit generosity (Newhouse 1994; Robinson, Gardner, and Luft 1993).

The reason for describing these sources of differences in preferences separately is that they may have quite different implications for judgments about the fairness of a set of health plan choices and the incentives for choosing among them. The idea that tastes for insurance may differ, and that individuals should be able to choose among a variety of plans that reflect these differences, seems to generate ambivalent reactions. On the one hand, most people appear to regard as inequitable an insurance system that makes individuals with more demand for generous benefits pay more simply because their existing health problems lead them to expect to use more medical care. Similarly, many people would regard a system of benefit choices that tended to segregate individuals with different income levels into plans with different levels of coverage as undesirable (see, for example, Fuchs 1993, Chapter 4, or LeGrand 1991, Chapters 6 and 7, for excellent discussions).

On the other hand, many would also regard as unfair a requirement that individuals who prefer different plans for reasons independent of their health be restricted to purchasing only a certain type of health insurance. If benefits are standardized, whose preferences about health insurance should be the "standard"? What mechanisms exist to assure that this desired standard is implemented? And what mechanisms will assure that, as medical technology progresses or individuals' preferences change, the standard plan will be updated accordingly?

This discussion suggests that standardization of benefits in Medicare should be tempered against other goals: some standardization but not complete standardization may be a desirable policy. Administrative costs and the need to establish plans that are large enough to pool risks effectively imply that a huge number of plans to accommodate every difference in taste for insurance benefits is not feasible. Most private employers offer only a limited number of plans, and many smaller employers offer only one (Newhouse 1996). But Medicare is easily a large enough program to offer some range of benefit choices. Before considering these options, the next section reviews some recent experiences of large employer-based health insurance purchasing groups. The experiences demonstrate some additional practical problems and opportunities that have arisen in the context of major private-sector reforms in health plan choices.

Private-Sector Experiences

In 1995, the University of California (UC) adopted a system of health plan choices for its employees modeled closely on the principles of managed competition developed by Alain Enthoven and others (Enthoven 1993). This system has several key features. First, UC standardized many features of the health plan choices offered to its employees. Eligible plans for employee purchase were required to cover "medically necessary" care and to offer identical benefits in terms of approximately 30 additional dimensions of covered services such as drugs, mental health services, and eyeglasses. Explicit diversity in benefits was allowed only in terms of insurance plan types: HMO, PPO, and FFS plans could be offered, as they had been previously. Second, UC switched to a fixed subsidy for employee purchase of a health plan regardless of choice. Previously, the employer subsidy was proportional to the plan premium, so that the employee paid some but not all of the additional expense of a more costly plan. Such fixed subsidies have also been proposed as Medicare reforms, to make beneficiaries more sensitive to the cost of alternative plans. The idea of a fixed subsidy is that a beneficiary would only be willing to pay another dollar in premiums if he or she believed that the more costly plan was worth another dollar in benefits.[5]

The UC reform had major effects on health plan choices (see Buchmueller and Feldstein 1996 for a more detailed discussion of the UC reform and its effects). With most dimensions of benefits standardized, employees found it much easier to compare plans. The plans only differed in price and type of insurance and in non-standardized "supply side" dimensions such as size of provider networks. Greater ease of comparison made employees' choices more sensitive to the more limited differences remaining among plans. In particular, employee choices became very sensitive to differences in price. For example, at UC Santa Cruz, a $5 higher premium caused 80 percent of employees enrolled in the traditionally more popular HMO to switch to an alternative HMO with the same benefits. In particular, the plan offered essentially the same healthcare providers. Following the adoption of this reform in 1994, UC healthcare expenditures declined (Enthoven 1996). Benefit standardization clearly increased competition among plans. Because the simultaneous change in employer contributions made employees much more sensitive to price differences, much of this enhanced competition occurred in the price of plans.

While standardization of benefits and fixed employer contributions have led to similar successes in limiting healthcare expenditures in many other firms, "managed competition" initiatives have sometimes faced greater difficulty in preserving a substantially more generous benefit option. For example, UC's most generous plan, in terms of the dimensions of provider choice and freedom from non-financial restraints on use of intensive services (dimensions that were not standardized), was a Prudential "high-option" fee-for-service plan. In the first year of UC's new system of plan choice, this plan had an out-of-pocket premium more than $70 higher per month compared to the HMO plans. More than 40 percent of prior enrollees switched out, leaving a smaller set of enrollees who were older and apparently had much higher healthcare costs than average employees. The result was a large premium increase and further massive disenrollment in 1995, and this "death spiral" cycle has continued. In 1997, the plan included only a few hundred older enrollees, with premiums of more than $700 per month (Richard Kronick personal communication).

Adverse selection into the most generous plan in a choice set, and offsetting favorable selection into less generous plans, has occurred often as private insurance purchasers have increased price competition among plans by standardizing many dimensions of benefits and increasing enrollee price sensitivity with changes in subsidies for purchasing plans. For example, the traditional fee-for-service plan at Stanford University experienced a similar death spiral when UC-like reforms were implemented there. In both of these cases, benefit managers regarded these plans as too generous to be a desired choice but perhaps faced too much employee opposition to eliminate them outright, and so little was done to try to stop the spirals. At other purchasing groups such as the Federal Employees Health Benefits Plan (Welch 1989) and at Harvard University, however, adverse selection spirals involving the most generous plan in a set of choices were not desired but have nonetheless been difficult to prevent. At Harvard, the spiral has occurred for a PPO alternative to HMOs in the setting of otherwise largely standardized benefits. Facing price incentives much like those at UC (but with somewhat less benefit standardization), younger and presumably healthier employees have switched out of the PPO plan (Cutler and Reber 1996).

Conclusions: Private-Sector Experiences with Benefit Standardization

By eliminating potentially confusing differences in many dimensions of plan benefits, standardization makes comparisons of benefits across plans much easier for potential enrollees, thereby leading to enrollee choices that are much more responsive to any remaining differences among plans. Standardization thus improves competition, presumably giving enrollees more value for their premiums. Because most private employers have implemented standardization along with reforms to increase enrollees' sensitivity to health plan prices, much of this enhanced competition has occurred in price. But price competition may encourage adverse selection in the plan that is most generous in retaining non-standardized dimensions, such as quality of provider networks or ease of obtaining intensive medical treatments. Because healthier individuals and individuals who have less taste for medical care for other reasons tend to place a lower value on the additional benefits, they will tend to choose lower-price plans over plans with more generous benefits. Standardization may worsen this selection problem by making comparisons easier.

Complete standardization of benefits would reduce the selection problem. If health plans were required to offer identical benefits in all dimensions, the price competition would be intense. But there would be no pressure for adverse selection, because competition in benefit generosity could not occur at all. Many employers (e.g., Stanford University) have limited selection problems by sharply limiting the dimensions in which plans can vary. But such sharp restrictions may create difficulties for an insurance purchaser with heterogeneous beneficiaries. Firm benefit managers also need to develop methods to help assure that the standard benefit package is the appropriate one for its beneficiaries. While benefit managers clearly have an interest in standardizing benefits in the way most preferred by employees,[6] little evidence exists regarding the performance of private or public purchasing groups in this role.

Allowing some choice of benefits could help ensure that benefits chosen more closely reflect enrollee preferences and may ease the problem of deciding which benefit plan is right. But because standardization improves competition, partial standardization of benefits may significantly worsen the adverse selection problem, possibly resulting in the elimination of the most generous type of plan that was intended to be available. This problem is likely to be particularly acute when competition in price rather than benefits is encouraged. Beneficiary subsidies for health insurance purchase that increase with health plan premiums, as in the Federal Employees Health Benefits Plan, would be expected to encourage more competition in benefits than the fixed subsidies regardless of plan choice. Although increasing subsidies presumably reduces the adverse selection pressures if benefits are not fully standardized, they will also tend to increase healthcare costs because employees do not face the full additional price of a plan with more generous benefits.

MEDICARE BENEFIT CHOICES TODAY

This section considers the choices available to Medicare beneficiaries in light of the issues and tradeoffs in benefit design considered in the previous section. Medicare beneficiaries can choose between coverage in "traditional" Medicare—essentially a fee-for-service insurance system, with or without a supplemental policy to cover the gaps in Medicare benefits—and enrollment in an increasingly broad range of alternative insurance plans. The Balanced Budget Act of 1997 broadened this range of insurance choices considerably, to allow not only Medicare HMOs but also preferred-provider plans, triple-option plans, medical savings accounts, and other innovative types of insurance. While benefits in traditional Medicare may appear to be completely standardized, the availability of a range of supplemental insurance options leads to important benefit choices even without considering managed care and other new options. The first part of this section considers diversity within traditional Medicare, and the second part considers choices between traditional Medicare and managed care alternatives.

Diversity in Traditional Medicare

Traditional Medicare consists of a standard set of benefits for all enrollees. Medicare hospital insurance (Part A) is an entitlement program financed by payroll taxes. Beneficiaries are responsible for an initial deductible (roughly equal to the cost of one hospital day) and are also responsible for partial and eventually complete copayments for very long hospital stays. Medicare hospital insurance also provides coverage for alternatives to hospitalization, including home health benefits, short-term skilled nursing facility benefits after hospitalization, and hospice benefits. Medicare Part B insurance is a voluntary program that beneficiaries can join or drop on a monthly basis. Part B insurance is largely financed by general revenues, but beneficiaries are required to pay a premium equal to around one-fourth of the program costs ($43.80 per month in 1998). Part B provides coverage for physician services, ambulatory health care, durable medical equipment, and other non-hospital services. Because Part B benefits are heavily subsidized, and because the alternative in traditional Medicare is no coverage for physician or ambulatory care, around 95 percent of the elderly in traditional Medicare are enrolled in Part B in any month. Approximately 99 percent of the elderly are enrolled in Part A. Even these figures probably understate actual coverage: because enrollment is allowed on a monthly basis, those elderly who decline coverage can get it relatively quickly if an illness arises.[7]

More choice exists among Medigap policies, which are private insurance policies that cover Medicare copayments and deductibles as well as some services not covered by Medicare. Medicare beneficiaries who do not qualify for Medicaid can obtain this additional coverage through two main types of Medigap policies: employer-provided plans (which are typically subsidized by a former employer), and individually-purchased plans.[8] Because the benefits of employer-provided Medigap are typically determined by an employer for all eligible beneficiaries, benefit choice and risk selection have not been major issues for these plans. Policies on choice and pricing in the individual Medigap insurance market illustrate important issues in benefit diversity and standardization.

Initially, the content and pricing of Medigap policies were only loosely regulated, leading to a proliferation of policy types. Considerable evidence exists that such proliferation resulted in poor consumer knowledge about available policies, leading to problems such as sales of duplicate policies. Profit levels were apparently high: the average "loss ratio" for these plans—benefit payouts divided by premiums—was well below 70 percent. While individual policies have relatively high administrative costs, these low loss ratios probably also reflected the lack of competition caused by information problems and plan diversity, as well as heavy spending by insurers to market these low-payout plans. Congress adopted the Baucus Amendments of 1980 to encourage states to establish minimum Medigap benefit requirements, set minimum loss ratios, and provide better information to purchasers about benefits. After the reforms, insurers continued to offer a variety of policies beyond the minimum package, so that gathering information on the price and benefits of alternative plans remained costly. Payout rates continued to be relatively low, and states had considerable difficulty in enforcing limits on insurer payout margins (Rice, McCall, and Boismier 1991).

Legislation in OBRA-90 addressed this problem by requiring new policies to consist of one of ten standard benefit packages. The packages were standardized in nine dimensions: coverage of "core" benefits (mainly Part A and Part B coinsurance, required of all plans),[9] Part A deductible coverage, Part B deductible coverage, coverage of Part B charges beyond the "allowed" Medicare fee charge,[10] coinsurance for some home health services not covered by Medicare, some home health visits beyond those covered by Medicare, preventive medical services, foreign travel, and prescription drug coverage. Thus, most of the allowed benefits for Medigap plans today involve coverage of copayments and deductibles for Medicare services, rather than coverage for additional types of medical care. The standardized Medigap drug benefits are of only limited generosity: the benefit provides 50 percent coinsurance after a $250 deductible, and the "low" option plan has an annual benefit of $1,250 while the "high" option plan has an annual benefit of $3,000.

Insurers are required to offer open enrollment in Medigap plans for all beneficiaries during their first six months of Medicare enrollment. Plans are not allowed to impose preexisting-condition exclusions for more than a six-month period, but they can refuse coverage after the open enrollment period, and they are allowed to "age adjust" premiums. OBRA-90 included a provision allowing Medigap insurers to offer "innovative benefits" so that the standards would not unduly retard innovation in insurance products. However, very few such plans have been adopted, and those that have typically only cover a particular service not included in the standard Medigap plan like drug and vision care (McCormack et al. 1996).

Table 6.2 summarizes takeup of individual Medigap plans in 1993 under this system of standardized benefits, along with changes in premiums in the plans between 1992 and 1994, in six states. McCormack et al. (1996) report that state insurers and consumers generally believe standardization has reduced uncertainty about plan comparisons, though some seniors still regard ten plan choices as confusing. Loss ratios (ratios of payouts to plan premiums) for individual policies increased from around 70 to 75 percent between 1990 and 1994, suggesting that price competition among plans has increased, that marketing and other administrative expenditures by plans have declined, or both.

As with standardization in employer plans, steps to make comparisons easier and thereby to increase competition among plans may also increase adverse selection pressures. Because individual Medigap purchases are not subsidized (that is, the beneficiary is responsible for the full price of the premium), and because the nature of Medigap benefits leaves plans little leeway in varying generosity within the standard choices,[11] one would expect price competition to be significantly greater after the OBRA-90 reforms.[12] If adverse selection is a problem, the difference in premiums between the most generous plan—the plan that would be expected to face the strongest adverse selection pressures—and the less generous alternatives will be greater than the actuarial value of the difference in premiums between the plans.

Determining actuarial differences between the standardized plans is not straightforward, because the plans differ in more than one dimension. However, in a careful effort to calculate the extent of adverse selection in the

Table 6.2 Standardized Medigap Plan Enrollment and Premiums

Medigap Plan Letter and Benefit Summary	Share of Plan Sales, 1994	Average Premiums, 1994	Change in Premiums 1992–94
B: Core benefits, Part A deductible	17.1%	$838	3%
C: Core benefits, Part A deductible, Part B deductible, SNF coinsurance, foreign healthcare	21.2	$908	4
D: Core benefits, Part A deductible, SNF coinsurance, foreign health care, home health	8.4	$872	5
F: Core benefits, Part A deductible, Part B deductible, SNF coinsurance, Part B excess charges ("low" option), foreign healthcare	29.7	$1,117	3
I: Core benefits, Part A deductible, SNF coinsurance, Part B excess charges ("high" option), home health, foreign health care, prescription drugs ("low" option)	5.9	$1,344	6
J: Core benefits, Part A deductible, Part B deductible, SNF coinsurance, Part B excess charges ("high" option), home health, foreign healthcare, prescription drugs ("high" option), preventive care	6.9	$1,811	17

Note: Core benefits include Part A hospital coinsurance for stays longer than 60 days, 365 additional "lifetime reserve" hospital days, Part B coinsurance, and blood deductibles. The prescription drug benefit consists of a 50 percent copayment after a $250 deductible, up to a maximum payment of $1,250 in the "low" option and $3,000 in the "high" option.

Source: McCormack et al. (1996), based on data from state insurance departments in Florida, Missouri, New York, South Carolina, Texas, and Washington.

most generous plan (Plan J), McCormack et al. (1996) estimate that $795 of this plan's $1,811 average premium in 1994 was the result of its relatively generous drug benefit. Because the actuarial cost of this benefit was only around $350 for an average elderly beneficiary, the extent of adverse selection into the most generous Medigap plan appears to be substantial. This plan has also experienced by far the most rapid premium growth since benefit standardization, increasing by 17 percent between 1992 and 1994. The low takeup rate of plans with drug benefits, despite the fact that none of these plans provide particularly generous drug coverage, is also consistent with adverse selection leading to suboptimal coverage rates. Despite the frequency with which illnesses may result in prescription drug use in the elderly, only 17 percent of the elderly with individual Medigap plans purchase a drug benefit.[13] In contrast, the drug coverage rate in the employer-provided plans is well over 50 percent. The employer-provided plans are typically purchased for larger groups and have subsidized premiums (reducing price competition), so that pressures for adverse selection are considerably lower.

Thus, Medicare's experience with Medigap standardization bears some similarities to the experiences of many private insurance purchasers with standardization of health plan choices for their nonelderly employees. Standardization appears to have increased price competition substantially, leading to reductions in loss ratios and apparently less confusion about choices and more satisfaction with Medigap among Medicare beneficiaries. However, the high prices and low enrollment rates in the most generous Medigap plan suggests that these changes have resulted in adverse selection problems, especially involving drug benefits. These adverse selection problems could be reduced through further restrictions in plan diversity; for example, many employers require a single drug benefit in all the plans offered to their employees. Reductions in adverse selection through further limitations on choices must be weighed against requiring beneficiaries to purchase benefits that they do not want. Indeed, some analysts have argued for more options to be included in the standard Medigap options, such as a catastrophic coverage benefit, or for such benefits to be required.[14]

In any event, the magnitude of adverse selection and choice problems in the Medigap market has been limited by the relatively small size of the supplemental benefits involved. The stakes are potentially much greater for the choice and selection problems involving Medicare managed care plans, and the other new plan options allowed in the Balanced Budget Act.

Diversity in Medicare Managed Care

Increasingly, Medicare beneficiaries are choosing an alternative to traditional Medicare and Medigap: enrollment in a managed care plan. This discussion focuses on the principal alternative to traditional Medicare as of 1998, "risk" HMOs, which are managed care plans that provide all services for the beneficiary for a fixed monthly payment.[15] All of the recent rapid growth in Medicare managed care has involved risk plans (PPRC 1997). The reimbursement that risk plans receive consists of a monthly payment from Medicare, the adjusted area per capita cost (AAPCC), and possibly an additional monthly premium assessed by the plan and paid by the beneficiary or the beneficiary's former employer. In 1997, the AAPCC payment was equal to 95 percent times the average Medicare expenditures for a "similar" enrollee in the beneficiary's county of residence, with "similar" defined on the basis of the enrollee's entitlement status (elderly, disabled, end-stage renal disease), age group, gender, Medicaid eligibility, and residence status (nursing home or community). Thus, the AAPCC payment has featured only limited risk adjustment, and the beneficiary premium (if any) must be the same for all enrollees. Risk plans must be approved by HCFA and are required to cover "medically necessary" care with at least the level of benefits in traditional Medicare.[16] Plans can offer additional benefits not covered by traditional Medicare, such as the benefits that may be included in Medigap plans.

The features of Medicare's 1998 system of plan choice differ in several important respects from the choice system in the Medigap market and in many private health insurance purchasing groups. First, though minimum benefits are required, Medicare HMO benefits are not standardized. To assist in health plan choice, HCFA produces "benefits comparison charts" modeled on those used by many other insurance purchasing groups (see Hoy, Wicks, and Forland 1996 for a more detailed description of methods used by purchasers to facilitate plan comparisons). The provision of such benefit information is mandated in the BBA. These charts report the additional HMO beneficiary premium (if any) and coverage of the following types of medical care: hospital care, physician care, skilled nursing care, home health care, emergency care (including urgent care outside the United States), preventive healthcare, dental care, outpatient drugs, mental health care, and whether the plan offers a "point of service" feature.

Such information is unquestionably helpful for making plan comparisons and probably has improved competition among plans in benefits offered. But Table 6.2 suggests that plans can differ in a large number of minor details within each of these benefit dimensions. Because these minor details can add up, understanding plan choices in Medicare is considerably more difficult than understanding the much more standardized systems just described for private insurance plans and for individual Medigap purchases. This choice system would be expected to lead to greater beneficiary uncertainty about actual coverage, greater effort and time costs to compare plans, and thus plan choices that are less responsive to actual differences in plans. The result may be less competition among HMO plans in benefits and price and perhaps relatively more direct advertising and other efforts to differentiate plans based on benefits than may be the case if benefits were standardized. On the other hand, lack of standardization allows more innovation in benefit design, and benefits included in managed care plans have changed considerably in recent years. Because managed care plans for Medicare beneficiaries are relatively new and untested products, such innovation may be particularly valuable now until the types of plans preferred by Medicare beneficiaries and the most important problems with implementing managed care plans for Medicare become clearer.

Second, Medicare's current system of plan choice directly limits price competition. The lowest premium that an HMO is allowed to charge for covering a Medicare beneficiary is determined by the AAPCC payment rate. A Medicare HMO may contract for a higher total premium with the additional amount paid by the beneficiary, but HMOs cannot contract to provide services at lower rates. This limits the price incentive facing Medicare beneficiaries for choosing between traditional Medicare and HMO plans. In effect, the AAPCC payment system for HMOs implies that Medicare, not the beneficiary, pays the 5 percent difference in premiums between traditional and managed care Medicare, if the beneficiary elects to enroll in traditional Medicare.[17]

Both of these features differ from the price competition in many private systems of health plan choice and in the individual Medigap market, and both probably limit price competition among plan choices. If beneficiaries had to pay the 5 percent difference between HMOs and traditional Medicare—which would have amounted to more than $200 per year in 1996— one could expect even more enrollment in HMOs, particularly by beneficiaries who placed relatively low value on the lack of restrictions on providers and treatments in traditional Medicare. Moreover, the "price floor" restricting price competition among managed care plans was binding for most HMOs in 1996 and 1997; the majority of Medicare HMO enrollees paid no HMO premiums. These restrictions on price competition suggest that if competition is occurring in health plan choices, it is likely to be occurring primarily in benefits. Once an HMO has reduced its beneficiary premium to zero, price competition is not possible; increasing generosity of benefits is the alternative way to compete for enrollees.

Moreover, the mechanism by which AAPCC payment rates are updated tends to support competition in benefit generosity. Except for risk adjusters, the AAPCC payment is not determined by the average cost of care for patients in the HMO; rather, it is determined by the average cost of care for area patients who are not enrolled in HMOs. Suppose that HMOs manage to attract more beneficiaries from traditional Medicare, either by offering more generous benefits or (if possible) lowering the beneficiary premium. If these beneficiaries are healthier than the average beneficiaries in traditional Medicare, then the average cost of a Medicare enrollee and hence the AAPCC will rise.[18] In turn, this higher payment rate would encourage the HMO to attract more beneficiaries (in particular, beneficiaries whose costs may have made them unprofitable at the previous payment rate), either by lowering premiums or by offering more generous benefits. This hypothesized "benefit spiral" with increasing HMO benefit generosity, increasing HMO enrollment, and increasing per capita Medicare costs is a very different outcome than the "death spiral" of decreasing availability of generous benefits that may occur with strong price competition.

With these features of Medicare benefit choices in mind, we briefly review some of the evidence on benefits and selection in HMOs versus traditional Medicare. As reported in Chapter 2, most studies find that HMOs experience favorable selection. For example, based on a detailed beneficiary survey, Brown et al. (1993) estimated that the expected costs of HMO enrollees, had they been in traditional Medicare, would have been approximately 83 percent as high as the costs of enrollees in traditional Medicare. The selection effects appear largest for new enrollees—as could be expected—and are smaller on average for enrollees who have been in HMOs for longer time periods.[19] Less evidence exists on changes over time in HMO benefits, enrollment, and selection. If competition among Medicare HMOs increases, do benefits become more generous and does favorable selection decline?

Table 6.3, which summarizes the measures of HMO benefits reported by HCFA, shows that HMO enrollees receive substantial additional benefits compared to traditional Medicare, especially in very recent years.[20] The table divides the supplemental HMO benefits into preventive care coverage, which is likely to be particularly valuable to healthy enrollees, and additional coverage of medical treatments, which is likely to be particularly valuable to beneficiaries with health problems requiring these treatments. In general, Medicare HMOs have provided substantial and increasingly generous benefits for preventive healthcare. Physical exams are covered for almost all HMO enrollees, and eye exams, ear exams, and immunizations are covered for most. These preventive benefits are likely to be particularly valuable to enrollees who do not have significant health problems, so that providing these benefits may be a way to attract relatively health enrollees.

Some types of treatment benefits provided by Medicare HMOs have also become more generous over time as well. For example, 70 percent of HMO enrollees in 1996 received supplemental drug benefits (up from 51

Table 6.3   Benefits in Medicare Risk HMOs, 1993–1996

	1993	1994	1995	1996
Number of risk plans	93	135	172	232
Enrollment (millions)	1.8	2.3	3.1	4.1
Average monthly beneficiary premium (basic plan)	$26.17	17.91	18.14	13.17
Preventive Benefits				
Physical exam	98%	97%	94%	97%
Immunizations	96	92	86	85
Health education	41	43	36	36
Eye exam	63	61	86	91
Ear exam	57	58	64	72
Other preventive care	16	27	30	25
Treatment Benefits				
Drug benefits	51%	49%	49%	70%
Dental coverage	13	20	25	32
Foot care	17	21	27	33
Prescription lenses	3	19	10	14
Hearing aid	1	15	3	3
Additional days of inpatient mental health care	0	0	0	0

Source: Author's tabulations from Medicare GHP data on "basic" benefits and premiums provided by the Office of Managed Care, Health Care Financing Administration, for December of each year. Premium and benefit statistics are weighted by plan enrollment.

percent in 1993), and one-third of enrollees were in plans that provided supplemental dental coverage and foot care (up from 13 percent and 17 percent in 1993, respectively). These supplemental benefits—especially drugs—are probably more attractive to beneficiaries with health problems.[21] HMOs have been more reluctant to offer other treatment benefits related to chronic illnesses, such as hearing aid coverage and mental health benefits. The absence of risk adjustment for beneficiaries who are likely to use such treatment benefits is probably an important explanation for the limited emergence of these kinds of supplemental benefits.

The additional cost of the supplemental benefits to enrollees is low and declining: average beneficiary premiums have declined from $26 to $13 per month between 1993 and 1996. Coupled with the fact that HMOs charge minimal copayments and deductibles and also provide considerable catastrophic insurance not available in Medicare, the rapid growth in Medicare HMOs is quite predictable. While HMOs have experienced favorable selection on average, at least some of the additional Medicare payments to HMOs are being translated into increasingly generous supplemental coverage.[22] Certainly, the lack of standardization does not seem to be causing any benefit "skimping" in HMOs, and while the favorable risk selection that exists implies higher than necessary costs to Medicare and is associated with concerns about how well HMOs cater to the needs of sicker beneficiaries, the selection does not appear to be worsening over time. In the Medicare market, unlike in other insurance markets, the risk selection "problem" is of favorable rather than adverse selection into plans, and rather than death spirals of generous plans, the rules and incentives within which Medicare HMOs operate have encouraged increasingly generous benefit packages. These benefit diversity outcomes differ substantially from the experiences of many private purchasers.

Further evidence on this topic comes from comparisons across geographic areas where AAPCC rates differ substantially and where multiple HMO choices are available. For example, Welch (1996) finds that Medicare HMO enrollment growth has been more rapid in areas with more generous AAPCC rates and with higher HMO penetration (and thus more competing HMO choices) in the non-elderly insurance market. His results suggest that both higher HMO payment rates and more competing HMOs in a market are associated with lower beneficiary premiums and more provision of supplemental benefits.

This discussion is somewhat speculative, because little evidence exists on how Medicare's reimbursement rules are influencing the dynamics of benefit offerings, patient selection, and healthcare costs. Though death spirals are clearly not occurring, many important questions remain unanswered. To what extent do different payment levels lead to different offerings of managed care benefits? How do the benefits offered change over time, as HMO payment rates and enrollment patterns change? How would risk adjustment affect the composition of supplementary benefits offered? Is the limited pressure for price competition and risk selection under Medicare's current choice system worth the higher healthcare costs resulting from the more generous benefits? Further evidence on these questions will be helpful for guiding reforms on benefit diversity in Medicare.

BENEFIT DIVERSITY IN MEDICARE HEALTH PLANS: POLICY OPTIONS

What changes in Medicare benefit design may help preserve diversity in Medicare managed care benefits while achieving other important goals such as promoting competition, encouraging cost-effective choices, and limiting selection problems? This section considers several reforms in benefit diversity in light of the preceding analysis of Medicare's current system of benefit choices.

Standardization of Benefits

Standardization of benefits is a key feature of benefit management in private firms today. Many firms standardize coverage requirements (e.g., types of services covered and amounts of patient payment liability), fewer standardize dimensions such as plan type (e.g., HMO versus PPO), and none have standardized "supply-side" features that affect the actual generosity of benefits offered such as financial incentives for providers, sizes of networks, and utilization review methods. Because these private reforms have typically been implemented in conjunction with reforms that make enrollees more sensitive to the price of their benefit choices, they may create strong adverse selection pressures in the most generous plan in the choice set. Medicare has had a similar experience, on a smaller scale, with standardization of Medigap benefits. Competition has increased and purchases of low-value Medigap coverage have fallen, but the Medigap plan with the most generous drug coverage is relatively expensive as a result of adverse selection. In both settings, making plan choice easier through standardization has limited purchases of more generous benefit options, partly because of selection problems.

Similarly, standardization of HMO benefits in Medicare would make plan comparisons easier and presumably improve competition among plans. At the extreme, requiring all potential Medicare insurers to offer a single kind of benefit plan would maximize competition as well as minimize problems of risk selection. The cost of such standardization is loss of diversity. Medicare beneficiaries are much more heterogeneous than the employees of most firms, and their preferences about health plans are also likely to be more heterogeneous. The political difficulty of specifying a single benefit package is one important obstacle to complete standardization. Moreover, standardization also discourages new and potentially more efficient or valuable innovations in healthcare delivery, and many innovations appear to be occurring now in Medicare HMO markets.

Alternatively, plans may be required to conform to a range of standardized benefit choices, analogous to the ten choices of Medigap plans available today. This option preserves some diversity in benefits, in principle supporting more innovation in plan design and allowing more enrollees to choose benefit plans they prefer. However, little innovation has occurred in Medigap benefits. Partial standardization may result in adverse selection in some plan options, which may in turn limit the availability and affordability of the most generous standard plans.

Design of Benefit Choices

Selection problems appear to be greatest when one benefit choice is clearly the most generous in all or most dimensions of benefits, such as Plan J in

Medigap. To address this problem, standardized plan alternatives could be designed so that they are not simply more or less generous in all dimensions. For example, suppose that two plan choices are allowed: a managed care plan that offers low copayments and deductibles with a restricted network of providers, and a catastrophic plan with a high deductible but no restrictions on services or providers. This set of choices may be stable even with price competition because the catastrophic plan will tend to attract the very healthy (because they expect to use few services) and the very ill (because they have the strongest preferences for few restrictions on providers and intensive treatments). In effect, the fact that the catastrophic plan is more generous once the high deductible has been met places a "safety valve" on the extent of risk selection between plans.[23] Indeed, one alternative plan choice that seems to be relatively stable in private firms is a "triple option" plan, which provides limited catastrophic coverage (with high copayment rates) outside of a provider network. Such a plan typically requires more out-of-pocket payments than an HMO, but the promise of more generous coverage in the rare event of a major illness appears to be enough to attract relatively risk averse but healthy enrollees as well as those with chronic illnesses.

Other examples of balancing generosity across dimensions may include pairing more generous prescription drug coverage with less generous home health or rehabilitation coverage, or pairing coverage outside the United States with less generous coverage of elective services in the United States. These allowances for "managed" diversity do not prevent adverse selection. Instead, plans with benefits that balance generosity in different dimensions will simply discourage the concentration of the healthiest and sickest beneficiaries in particular plans. It would also discourage plans from uniformly varying quality in the dimensions of benefits that cannot be precisely standardized.

Competition in Price versus Benefits

Greater standardization is likely to increase competition among available plans, and such competition may occur in cost or in benefit generosity. As the experience of private purchasing groups and the Medigap market have suggested, making beneficiaries financially responsible for a greater part of the cost differences among plan choices will encourage beneficiaries to choose plans whose additional benefits are worth their additional costs. The current limitations on the sensitivity of beneficiaries to cost differences between traditional fee-for-service without supplementary coverage and managed care Medicare—beneficiaries are not responsible for the 5 percent higher Medicare payments if they choose the traditional program—may have contributed to the relatively slow takeup of managed care plans in the past despite their additional benefits. Making beneficiaries responsible for the difference in premiums, as many private employers do, could probably increase enrollment in managed care plans substantially. On the other hand, Medicare savings from more cost-conscious plan choices must be weighed against the greater adverse selection pressures in traditional Medicare that would also result. Because the healthiest beneficiaries in traditional Medicare tend to value the additional freedom of provider choice the least, they would be most likely to switch plans.

Restrictions on the payments that managed care plans can receive in the AAPCC system also limit price competition: once their beneficiary premiums are zero, plans can attract more enrollees only by offering more generous benefits or higher quality services. This may encourage more generous benefit choices that are optimal. If more price competition were allowed—for example, if managed care plans were allowed to cover the beneficiary's Part B premium—then they would be less likely to offer additional benefits to attract enrollees. While such reforms may reduce Medicare expenditures, they would also create greater problems of adverse selection for plans that offer generous benefits. Encouragement of benefit competition rather than price competition through Medicare's choice system is probably a major reason why managed care plans with relatively generous benefits have emerged and prospered in the absence of any benefit standardization and why severe adverse risk selection problems and a decline in the generosity of available choices have not occurred.

Limits on price competition reduce risk selection among benefit choices but also encourage health plans to offer more generous benefits to attract enrollees. While limiting Medicare expenditure growth may be an important policy goal, there are many reasons to suspect that encouraging price competition in Medicare plan choices would create more serious problems of adverse selection and insufficient health insurance that has occurred when employers have implemented reforms to increase price competition. The Medicare population includes a much larger proportion of beneficiaries with chronic health impairments, and many beneficiaries have functional impairments that may make it more difficult for them to evaluate alternative plans effectively. The potential vulnerability of many Medicare beneficiaries argues for incremental reforms in the incentives for price and generosity competition in Medicare's choice system and for preservation of at least some limits on price competition. Clearly, however, the rules for pricing alternative benefit choices will become even more important with steps that increase health plan competition in price and benefits, including standardization of benefits.

Other Considerations Affecting Benefit Design

Other Medicare reforms may have important effects on the desirability of a particular system of benefit choices. For example, adoption of a system of risk adjustment would be expected to reduce selection pressures. However, restrictions on price competition already limit selection pressures in Medicare's choice system, and thus risk adjustment may make reforms to increase price competition more desirable. Risk adjustment would also change the nature of benefit competition among HMOs. Benefits preferred by individuals with health problems included in the adjustments would become more favorable for plans to provide, and benefits preferred by individuals without such health problems would become less favorable. This change could tilt Medicare HMO benefits away from a heavy emphasis on preventive care and other coverage preferred by relatively healthy beneficiaries, making healthy Medicare beneficiaries relatively worse off but sicker ones potentially better off. Unlike benefit standardization and other steps to facilitate comparisons between plans, however, risk adjustment would not directly affect the extent of competition among health plans.

Another proposed Medicare financing reform, a reduction in managed care payment rates (especially for new HMO enrollees), would lead to reduced generosity of supplemental HMO benefits. The reduction in benefit generosity would tend to reduce HMO enrollment and perhaps would tend to increase favorable selection into HMOs. This reform would not affect the extent of competition, except to the extent that it reduced the number of HMO plans offered. These examples demonstrate how financing reforms not directly related to benefit generosity may have important effects on the benefits offered by health plans in Medicare.

Reforms that provide additional information about plans to beneficiaries would increase competition, to the extent that they facilitate comparison of plans. Indeed, the principal motivation for requiring standard benefit designs is to reduce beneficiary costs and uncertainty for comparing plans. In the individual Medigap market, beneficiaries need to know only the letter of a plan to understand its coverage. Managed care plans involve a substantially greater range of benefits than Medigap plans, including benefits that cannot easily be standardized such as the extent of provider networks. Thus, even if many dimensions of benefits are standardized and a limited number of options are offered, it is likely that information problems will remain. Features of plan "quality" that cannot easily be standardized will be difficult to incorporate in informational materials distributed to beneficiaries. These include descriptions of participating providers as well as process, outcome, and satisfaction measures that provide evidence on the access to and quality of medical treatments covered by the plan. Thus, increasing competition through reforms in benefit design is just one component of increasing competition among health plans.

KEY QUESTIONS FOR BENEFIT DIVERSITY

Benefit design, including such issues as standardization and diversity of benefit choices and the systems of financial incentives and information in which such choices occur, is a difficult issue for Medicare reform. While benefit standardization has many advantages, relatively little is known about which benefits or choices of benefits would be most desirable for the diverse Medicare population and which sets of choices will best address the problems of selection and competition in Medicare's distinctive system. These issues have not been completely resolved even in private firms and other purchasing groups that already have extensive experience with standardization of health plan benefits and that have undertaken fundamental reforms in health plan choice systems. Nonetheless, changes in Medicare's benefit choice system are an important consideration for Medicare reform. Even doing nothing about benefit choices will contribute to complexities elsewhere in the management of Medicare benefits, such as in regulation of increasing plan costs, risk adjustment, and the provision of information for effective competition among plans.

This chapter has considered several major issues involving benefit diversity in Medicare, which are summarized here.

Should benefits be standardized? Standardization would make comparisons across plans easier and would increase competition. Complete standardization would also minimize opportunities for risk selection among plans. But standardization has costs: the preferences of Medicare beneficiaries for health insurance differ substantially, and defining a single required set of benefits is a difficult political issue. Standardizing a set of benefit choices is one way to balance these concerns. The benefits of limited plan diversity were the principal motivation for the standardization of a range of Medigap plan choices in 1990. But standardization of a range of benefit choices also has costs: risk segmentation may be greater than in cases where benefits are less standardized, and only allowing a range of standardized benefits may limit innovation in the design of Medicare benefits.

If benefits are standardized, which health plan choices should be offered? Offering standardized choices of plans that are uniformly more or less generous may lead to significant adverse selection problems, even a death spiral of worsening selection and increasing premiums in the most generous plan. Limiting differences in generosity among standardized plan choices—for example, by designing choices so that no plan is uniformly more generous in all dimensions—could limit the extent of such selection problems at the cost of restricting one dimension of choice (the level of coverage).

Should price competition among benefit choices be encouraged? The extent to which risk selection would occur with any set of benefit choices depends on the extent to which the plans are encouraged to compete in price versus benefit generosity. Medicare's current payment system for managed care plans limits risk selection because it limits price competition. The greater price competition featured in many private health insurance purchasing groups provides stronger incentives to limit benefit generosity and thus healthcare costs and also encourages more risk selection if benefits are not fully standardized. Limited price competition among standardized plans is one method of balancing these concerns. For example, plan premiums could be allowed to vary over a limited range, and beneficiaries could be responsible for some but not all of the differences in premiums for plans with different benefits.

NOTES

1. We thank Rick Kronick, Joy de Beyer, and participants in the Commonwealth Fund's "Risk Adjustment Is Not Enough: Strategies to Limit Risk Selection in the Medicare Program," April 3, 1997 conference for useful discussions and helpful comments; Dominic Allocco for outstanding research assistance; and the Commonwealth Fund and the National Institute on Aging for financial support. All errors are our own.
2. Economists typically refer to this as the "adverse selection" problem, though risk selection can be favorable or adverse.
3. While many economic analyses have considered the willingness of employees and others to pay for more generous benefits, these studies have primarily focused on average willingness to pay rather than on the variations in willingness to pay in a population. If preferences differ, average willingness to pay is not a very good guide to the desirable diversity of benefits.
4. Mitigating this difference is the fact that any given amount of unpredictability about medical expenditures will be viewed more unfavorably by a lower-income individual; someone with a family income of $29,000 will face relatively less disruption in lifestyle from a medical expenditure of $2,000 than someone with a family income of $18,000. However, in managed care plans with low out-of-pocket payments, they may have quite different preferences about the size of provider networks or how the plan determines "medically necessary" treatments.
5. Because employer-paid premiums are tax deductible, this system still involves a "tax wedge" determined by their tax rate t: employees value $1 in premium contributions the same as $(1 - t)$ in earnings. Nonetheless, this type of reform would be expected to make beneficiaries much more sensitive

to the price of their benefit choices compared to the system of proportional subsidies.

6. That is, if a firm implements a standardized benefit package that employees do not like, they may move to other firms that offer the same total compensation with a more desirable package of health insurance, wages, and other fringe benefits. However, there are considerable costs to switching jobs for most employees, and even though health insurance is a major employment benefit, it is only one of many dimensions that employees evaluate in choosing a job. Health benefits may have to differ substantially from an employee's preferred package to lead to a switch. As a result, idiosyncratic historical experiences in how benefit standardization occurred may have an important effect on plan choices that actually emerge. For example, even though they have relatively similar characteristics and presumably similar preferences about benefits, in 1996 UC employees had relatively high enrollment rates in PPO plans, Harvard employees primarily used HMO plans, and more Stanford employees were enrolled in "triple option" plans.

7. Beneficiaries enrolled in Medicare HMOs must also pay the Part B premium.

8. "Individual" plans may also be marketed through groups such as AARP. However, participation is voluntary and not subsidized.

9. Part B coinsurance coverage for outpatient mental health care has been somewhat unclear: Medicare copayments for such services are 50 percent, not 20 percent, and plans have interpreted their liability differently (i.e., coverage of 20 percent versus 50 percent of fees).

10. While the Medicare fee schedule has reduced "balance billing" of additional charges by physicians, hospital outpatient departments have been allowed to bill beneficiaries for 20 percent of actual charges, not 20 percent of Medicare allowed charges. Thus, this benefit has been quite valuable. The "low" option plan covers 80 percent of the additional charges, and the "high" option plan covers all the additional charges.

11. Because these are add-ons to a fee-for-service plan, most of the dimensions of benefits involve supplementing copayments, deductibles, and maximum payment limits in traditional Medicare. While "managed care" benefits with restrictions on providers and use exist for drugs and nursing home care exists for the non-elderly, they are not allowed in the standardized benefit packages and have not been offered as "innovations." Thus, there is little room for product differentiation within the ten standardized categories.

12. McCormack et al. (1996) report that more carriers are adopting age-adjusted premiums, also suggesting that competition and selection have increased.

13. Of course, because Medigap insurers may employ underwriting, many beneficiaries may like to purchase plans with drug coverage but are rejected by the insurers.

14. Virtually all dimensions of the standardized Medigap plans involve limited benefits, so that catastrophic expenditures for drugs, hospital care, nursing home care, and home health care are not covered. An optional standardized catastrophic coverage plan is likely to face significant adverse selection

problems for the reasons described in the text, and many beneficiaries may oppose a required catastrophic benefit that they have to pay for, as the Catastrophic Coverage Act of 1989 demonstrated. Wisconsin, one of three "waiver" states exempted from OBRA-90 because it had passed its own standardization program previously, began offering a "catastrophic" drug coverage above an annual deductible of $6,250 (the level of out-of-pocket drug expenditures when the high-option drug benefit is exhausted) as part of its Medigap drug option. Takeup of this option has been limited.

15. Other forms of managed care contracts that were allowed in Medicare prior to the Balanced Budget Act include "cost" HMOs (HMO plans that are reimbursed just like providers in "traditional" Medicare, with similar implications for selection) and healthcare prepayment plans (HCPPs, which are like cost HMOs for Part A services only), and largely experimental forms such as social HMOs (a limited number of HMOs that provide medical care plus additional integrated support services for seniors).

16. Substantial copayments and deductibles for HMO services are prohibited under provisions of the HMO Act.

17. Of course there are substantial premium differences between most HMOs and traditional Medicare fee-for-service plus a Medigap policy (see Chapter 4). But beneficiaries without supplementary coverage would pay the same Part B premium in Medicare fee-for-service or a zero premium HMO (although would obviously face potentially large copayments and deductibles in fee-for-service that HMOs would cover).

18. In other words, if the HMO enrollees are healthier on average than traditional Medicare enrollees, the "marginal" beneficiary switching from traditional Medicare to the HMO will tend to be relatively healthy compared to the remaining traditional Medicare beneficiaries but relatively ill compared to the existing HMO beneficiaries. The switch will tend to raise the average cost in both the HMO and in traditional Medicare, even if the overall average cost for all beneficiaries is unchanged, and AAPCC payments will rise. On the other hand, HMO diffusion could help reduce overall Medicare costs if HMOs do practice a less costly style of medicine, and if this effect "spills over" into the treatment of traditional Medicare patients.

19. Evidence on this question is limited in large part because of the limited information available on the health and medical care of beneficiaries in HMOs. Studies comparing prior-year expenditures of beneficiaries who join HMOs versus those who stay in traditional Medicare typically find much larger differences in expected expenditures, but beneficiaries are much more likely to switch plans when they are not in the midst of an illness, and the differences appear to diminish substantially over time.

20. Many Medicare experts at HCFA and elsewhere have questioned the accuracy of the benefits reported by Medicare HMOs. Here, we focus on a qualitative interpretation of the benefit data; it seems clear that many supplemental benefits are offered and that, at least through 1996, the supplemental benefits were not declining. Improving the quality of supple-

mental benefit data reporting is an important policy concern as Medicare+ Choice options expand.

21. The exception may be preventive health benefits, which are probably more valuable to beneficiaries who do not expect to see their provider for treatment of an existing health problem anyway. We return to this issue shortly.

22. The HCFA "benefits comparison charts," which do provide specific information on some dimensions of HMO benefits, suggest that these benefits are generally not skimpy, especially in areas with many competing health plans such as Arizona and Northern California. Moreover, the vast majority of Medicare beneficiaries in HMOs appear to be satisfied with the care received in their plan (Nelson et al. 1997).

23. Keeler et al. (1996) and Eichner, McClellan, and Wise (1997) discuss the "safety valve" effect in more detail.

REFERENCES

Brown, R., J. Bergeron, D. Clement, J. Hill, and S. Retchin. 1993. "The Medicare Risk Program for HMOs—Final Summary Report on Findings from the Evaluation." Report submitted to the Department of Health and Human Services. Princeton, NJ: Mathematica Policy Research Inc.

Buchmueller, T., and P. Feldstein. 1996. "Consumers' Sensitivity to Health Plan Premiums: Evidence from a Natural Experiment in California." *Health Affairs* 15 (1): 143–51.

Chakraborty, G., R. Ettenson, and G. Gaeth. 1994. "How Consumers Choose Health Insurance." *Journal of Health Care Marketing* 14: 21–33.

Cutler, D., and S. Reber. 1996. "Paying for Health Insurance: The Tradeoff Between Competition and Adverse Selection." Cambridge: NBER working paper.

Eichner, M., M. McClellan, and D. Wise. 1997. "Health Persistence and the Feasibility of Medical Savings Accounts." In *Tax Policy and the Economy, Vol. 11*, edited by J. Poterba, 91–128. Cambridge: MIT Press.

Enthoven, A. 1993. "The History and Principles of Managed Competition." *Health Affairs* 12 (Suppl.): 24–48.

Enthoven, A. 1996. "Managed Competition and California's Health Care Economy." *Health Affairs* 15 (Spring): 39–57.

Fuchs, V. 1993. *The Future of Health Policy*. Cambridge: Harvard University Press.

Garber, A., and C. Phelps. 1997. "Economic Foundations of Cost-Effectiveness Analysis." *Journal of Health Economics* 16 (1): 1–31.

Hoy, E., E. Wicks, and R. Forland. 1996. "Best Practices for Structuring and Facilitating Consumer Choice of Health Plans." In *Improving the Medicare Market*, edited by S. Jones and M. E. Lewin, 159–94. Washington, DC: National Academy Press.

Keeler, E., J. Malkin, D. Goldman, and J. Buchanan. 1996. "Can Medical Savings Accounts for the Nonelderly Reduce Health Care Costs?" *Journal of the American Medical Association* 275 (21): 1666–71.

LeGrand, J. 1991. *Equity and Choice*. London: HarperCollins.

Litzenberger, R., and E. Ronn. 1986. "A Utility-Based Model of Common Stick Price Movements." *Journal of Finance* 15: 67–92.

McCormack, L., P. Fox, T. Rice, and M. Graham. 1996. "Medigap Reform Legislation of 1990: Have the Objectives Been Met?" *Health Care Financing Review* 18 (1): 157–74.

Nelson, L., R. Brown, M. Gold, A. Ciemnecki, and E. Docteur. 1997. "Access to Care in Medicare HMOs." *Health Affairs* 16 (2): 148–63.

Newhouse, J. 1994. "Patients at Risk: Health Reform and Risk Adjustment." *Health Affairs* 13 (1): 132–46.

Newhouse, J. 1996. "Reimbursing Health Plans and Health Providers: Efficiency in Production versus Selection." *Journal of Economic Literature* 34 (3): 1236–63.

Newhouse, J. P., W. G. Manning, E. B. Keeler, and E. M. Sloss. 1989. "Adjusting Capitation Rates Using Objective Health Measures and Prior Utilization." *Health Care Financing Review* 10 (3): 41–54.

Physician Payment Review Commission. 1997. *Annual Report to Congress.* Washington, DC.

Rice, T., N. McCall, and J. Boismier. 1991. "The Effectiveness of Consumer Choice in the Medicare Supplemental Health Insurance Market." *Health Services Research* 26: 223–46.

Robinson, J., L. Gardner, and H. Luft. 1993. "Health Plan Switching in Anticipation of Increased Medical Care Utilization." *Medical Care* 31 (1): 43–51.

Szpiro, G. 1986. "Measuring Risk Aversion: An Alternative Approach." *Review of Economics and Statistics* 68 (1): 156–59.

Welch, W. P. 1989. "Restructuring the Federal Employees Health Benefits Program: The Private Sector Option." *Inquiry* 26 (3): 321–34.

Welch, W. P. 1996. "Growth in HMO Share of the Medicare Market: 1989–1994." *Health Affairs* 15 (3): 201–14.

7

Stronger Oversight and Additional Regulation of Plans

Gerard Anderson

One method of limiting the extent of risk selection in the Medicare program is for the federal government to credential or regulate healthcare plans. By requiring all managed care plans to become credentialed, the government can ensure that each plan will provide a relatively similar product, offer access to a similar set of providers, and provide a similar level of quality of service. By using credentialing to restrict the number of health plans in a geographic area, the federal government can reduce the extent of risk selection if high-risk individuals are more evenly distributed across relatively few plans. By regulating health plan behavior, the government can ensure that health plans will not take specific actions to encourage risk selection and if health plans take specific actions, then the government can sanction them.

This chapter will focus on individuals with chronic illnesses for several reasons. First, without adequate risk adjustment, chronically ill individuals are especially vulnerable in a managed care environment. The 99 million Americans with one or more chronic illnesses were estimated to cost $470 billion in 1995 (Hoffman, Rice, and Sung 1996). On a per capita basis, individuals with two or more chronic illnesses were 5.7 times more expensive than individuals with only an acute condition (Hoffman, Rice, and Sung 1996). Second, the chronically ill utilize a somewhat different configuration of services than the acutely ill, providing managed care plans an opportunity to take actions to discourage the enrollment of the more expensive chronically ill individuals (Ireys et al. 1997). This chapter is organized into three sections. The first section describes the cost of providing services to chronically ill individuals and the mix of services they utilize. It shows that chronically ill individuals use certain medical care at much higher rates. These are services that managed care plans could target to achieve favorable selection. The second section examines legislative and regulatory actions undertaken by state governments to regulate or credential managed care plans. The focus in this section will be on state provisions that could help reduce risk selection. The section does not discuss alternative payment methods that some states have implemented to explicitly adjust payment rates to managed care plans. Finally, in the third section, we will use the information presented in sections one and two to develop specific recommendations that the federal government should consider for the Medicare program.

WHY THE CHRONICALLY ILL MAY BE A TARGET FOR RISK SELECTION

Individuals with chronic illnesses are especially vulnerable in a managed care environment without adequate risk adjusters. Numerous studies have shown that the aggregate cost of chronic illnesses, the costs of specific chronic illnesses and the per capita costs of providing services to individuals with chronic illnesses are substantial. Studies have found that children with chronic illnesses are five to 20 times more expensive than children without chronic illnesses and that the elderly with chronic illnesses have higher per capita costs (Neff and Anderson 1995; Anderson et al. 1990).

In Table 7.1, we compute per capita expenditures from a 5 percent random national sample of aged Medicare beneficiaries (as distinct from disabled or end-stage renal disease Medicare beneficiaries). We compare the expenditures per capita for aged Medicare beneficiaries with one of ten selected chronic illnesses to all aged Medicare beneficiaries. Per capita expenditures by the Medicare program for individuals with chronic illnesses are two to five times more than for the "average" Medicare beneficiary. Medicare beneficiaries with at least one of these ten diagnoses represented 42 percent of all Medicare beneficiaries and accounted for 80 percent of Medicare spending in 1992–93. It is important to recognize that some of these expenditures were for services that may be unrelated to the Medicare beneficiary's chronic condition.

Table 7.2 presents information on service use for these aged chronically ill Medicare beneficiaries. We found that Medicare beneficiaries with one of the ten chronic illnesses were more likely than all Medicare benefi-

Table 7.1 Expenditures Per Capita for Aged Medicare Beneficiaries, 1992–1993

Diagnostic Category	Expenditure Per Capita	Ratio of Expenditure Per Capita to Aged Medicare Beneficiaries
Parkinson's disease	$11,598	4.6
Colon cancer	10,221	4.1
Lung cancer	8,616	3.5
Stroke	8,571	3.3
Liver cirrhosis	8,468	3.3
Chronic obstructive pulmonary disease	8,106	3.2
Ischemic heart disease	6,344	2.6
Alzheimer's	6,094	2.4
Diabetes	4,837	1.9
Arthritis	4,186	1.7
All aged Medicare beneficiaries	2,541	1.0

Source: Based on analyses of 1992 Medicare Standard Analytic Files.

ciaries to utilize home health services. The greater use of other services by aged chronically ill Medicare beneficiaries was more dependent on the specific medical condition. For example, Medicare beneficiaries with chronic obstructive pulmonary disease (COPD) used durable medical equipment at a much higher rate than beneficiaries with other chronic conditions. Much of the difference in the use of services by chronically ill Medicare beneficiaries compared to all Medicare beneficiaries is in their use of specialists (data not shown). For example, Medicare beneficiaries with Alzheimer's disease are much more likely to see psychiatrists and psychologists, beneficiaries with COPD to see pulmonologists, and beneficiaries with ischemic heart disease to see cardiovascular surgeons.

The greater reliance on certain services and specialists by the chronically ill Medicare beneficiaries is another reason why there is a need for risk adjustment in Medicare programs. In the absence of adequate risk adjusters, expected higher per capita expenditures provide an incentive for managed care plans not to enroll chronically ill individuals. For managed care organizations attempting to discourage the enrollment of the chronically ill, their dependence on certain types of providers gives managed care plans an easy way to structure the delivery system to discourage their enrollment. By increasing the queue for services, by making access to the services more difficult (e.g., increasing travel times), or by attracting less qualified providers, the managed care plan can be less attractive to the chronically ill who need these services.

Table 7.2 Ratio of Average Payment for Aged Medicare Beneficiaries with Chronic Conditions to All Medicare Beneficiaries, by Type of Service, 1992–1993

Chronic Condition	All Services	Inpatient	Outpatient	Part B	Durable Medical Equipment	Home Health
Alzheimer's	2.3	2.5	1.6	2.0	4.7	4.8
Chronic obstructive pulmonary disease	3.2	3.6	1.9	2.8	7.2	9.5
Ischemic heart disease	2.4	2.7	1.9	2.2	1.9	2.4
Diabetes	1.9	1.9	1.9	1.9	1.9	1.9
Lung cancer	3.3	3.8	2.9	2.7	3.0	4.2
Arthritis	1.6	1.5	1.5	1.6	1.3	3.5
Stroke	3.3	3.7	2.4	2.7	3.9	5.8
Cirrhosis	3.6	4.2	2.8	2.8	2.3	6.0
Colon cancer	3.8	4.2	3.0	3.3	2.2	4.4
Parkinson's disease	2.2	2.3	1.8	2.0	1.9	9.1

Source: Based on analyses of 1992 Medicare Standard Analytic Files.

As Kronick and de Beyer argue in Chapter 2, "the choice of healthcare providers available through a plan and the places where that care is provided can have a powerful effect on who enrolls." Because access to specialty physicians or to services such as durable medical equipment or home health is difficult, some chronically ill individuals may choose not to enroll in a managed care plan or may choose to disenroll once they encounter difficulty accessing these services. Individuals without chronic illnesses, however, are unlikely to need or utilize many of these services. Therefore, it may be possible for some managed care plans to limit access to these services without seriously affecting their overall enrollment levels. This is one way that healthcare plans could achieve favorable selection. The next section reviews legislative and regulatory initiatives taken by states that have potential to reduce the vulnerability of chronically ill to risk selection.

STATE LEGISLATION AND REGULATION OF MANAGED CARE PLANS

Most of the regulatory and legislative activity involving managed care has occurred at the state level. For this reason we turn to the states for suggestions about regulatory and legislative options that the Medicare program should consider to reduce the amount of risk selection. In 1996, state legislatures introduced more than 400 legislative proposals to regulate the managed care industry—twice as many as in 1995 and four times as many as in

1994 (Azevedo 1996). In 1996, state legislatures passed 56 bills in 35 states regulating the actions of managed care plans (Bodenheimer 1996). Although the level of interest in regulating managed care varies considerably from state to state, nearly all states have passed some form of legislation regulating managed care plans.

In order to investigate the types of legislation that states are enacting, state legislation governing managed care was reviewed. The legislation was identified by consulting an online service, LEXIS/NEXIS, and searching on the following key words: "managed care" or "health maintenance organization." A summary of the legislative activity is presented in Table 7.3. Table 7.4 shows the types of legislation passed by each state as of November 1997.

Most of the state legislation to regulate managed care plans can be categorized into four general categories: (1) access to care; (2) quality of care; (3) financing; and (4) consumer protection (Table 7.3). This section summarizes the proposed and enacted state legislation in order to identify common themes and regulatory approaches. Given the wide range of proposed and enacted legislation, no attempt is made to be comprehensive. Rather, the general approaches taken by states will be illustrated by examples from one or more states. The focus will be on state provisions that could reduce the amount of risk selection in managed care plans.

Access to Care

Numerous newspaper and other media reports have noted that some managed care plans have denied the chronically ill access to specialty providers and other services. Most states have responded to these concerns with legislation designed to ensure access to health plans and to certain types of providers.

Many states do not allow managed care plans to cancel or refuse to renew an individual solely on the basis of his or her health status. For example, Delaware law states, "No health maintenance organization may cancel or refuse the enrollment of an enrollee solely on the basis of the enrollee's health" (16 Del. C. 1996). Other states are more specific and protect individuals with a particular illness, probably in response to one or more instances in which a person was denied access to insurance. Some states have legislation prohibiting managed care plans from imposing exclusions on individuals with preexisting conditions. For example, managed care plans in North Carolina are required to enroll applicants with sickle cell trait or hemoglobin C trait (NC Gen. Stat. 1996). Other states allow managed care plans to impose preexisting conditions exclusions only if certain requirements are met.

Table 7.3   State Approaches to Managed Care Legislation, Regulation, and Credentialing

I. Access to Care

Open Enrollment

- Marketing restrictions
- Direct access to specific specialist
- Access to specific services
- Coverage of experimental treatments
- No preexisting condition exclusions
- Coverage of emergency care
- Acceptance of any willing provider
- Mandated hours of services for Medicaid plans

II. Quality of Care

- Licensing requirements
- Medical audit requirements
- Credentialing requirements
- Quality requirements

III. Financing

- Capitalization requirements
- Financial requirements
- Reserves/deposits requirements
- Disclosure of financial arrangements/no gag rules

IV. Consumer Protection

- Evidence of coverage provided
- Confidentiality of medical information requirements
- Complaint/grievance system

By late 1997, 22 states had enacted laws allowing health plan members either direct access to a particular specialist or the choice of a specialist as a primary care provider. In 1987, Florida became the first state to pass a direct access law by allowing chiropractors to be designated as primary care providers. Since the passage of the Florida law, most of the direct access legislation has focused on ensuring women direct access to obstetricians, gynecologists, or other women's healthcare providers. Our review of the legislation indicates that as of November 1997, at least 19 states had passed laws ensuring women direct access to obstetricians/gynecologists. States have also granted health plan members direct access to specific specialists, such as optometrists or ophthalmologists in Arkansas (Ark. Stat. Ann. 1995), dermatologists in Georgia (O.C.G.A. 1995), and chiropractors in Kentucky (KRS 1996).

Table 7.4   State Legislation Indicators Monitoring Managed Care

	1	2	3	4	5	6	7	8	9	10	11	12	13	14	15
AL			x				x	x	x		x		x	x	x
AK			x		12			x	x		x		x	x	x
AZ								x	x	x					x
AR	x	x	x	x*				x	x	x	x		x	x	x
CA			x	*		x		x	x	x	x	x	x	x	x
CO	x	x	x		12		x	x	x		x	x	x	x	x
CT			x	x		x		x	x	x			x	x	x
DE			x				x	x	x	x	x	x		x	
DC			x		2			x	x	x	x	x	x	x	x
FL	x	x	x	*	123	x		x	x	x	x	x	x	x	x
GA			x	x*	1	x	x	x	x	x	x	x	x	x	x
HI			x		1	x		x	x	x	x		x	x	x
ID	x	x	x	x*	12		x	x	x	x	x		x	x	x
IL	x	x	x		124	x		x	x	x	x		x	x	x
IN		x	x		124	x	x	x	x	x	x	x	x	x	x
IA	x		x		12			x	x	x	x		x	x	x
KS	x				1			x	x	x	x		x	x	x
KY	x		x	*	123		x	x	x	x	x		x	x	x
LA			x	x			x	x	x	x	x		x	x	x
ME	x	x	x	x*	124			x	x	x	x	x	x	x	x
MD			x	x	14	x		x	x	x	x	x	x	x	x
MA	x		x		13	x		x	x			x	x	x	
MI	x	x	x	x	24		x	x	x	x	x	x	x	x	x
MN			x	x	1	x	x	x	x		x	x	x		x
MS				x	1	x	x	x	x	x	x		x	x	x

Continued

Table 7.4 (continued)

	1	2	3	4	5	6	7	8	9	10	11	12	13	14	15
MO			x	x	23	x	x	x	x	x	x	x	x	x	x
MT			x				x	x	x		x		x	x	x
NE			x					x	x	x	x		x	x	x
NV	x		x		124			x	x		x		x		x
NH	x		x		13		x	x	x		x	x	x		x
NJ	x	x	x	x*	123		x	x	x	x	x		x	x	x
NM			x		12		x	x	x	x	x		x	x	x
NY			x		1			x	x	x	x	x	x	x	x
NC			x	x	124	x	x	x	x	x	x		x	x	x
ND			x		12			x	x	x	x		x	x	x
OH	x	x	x		12			x	x	x	x		x	x	x
OK			x		1			x		x	x	x	x		x
OR				x*			x	x		x		x		x	x
PA			x		2			x	x	x	x				x
RI		x	x		1234			x	x	x	x	x	x	x	x
SC			x		1			x	x	x	x		x	x	x
SD			x		12		x	x	x	x	x		x	x	x
TN			x		123			x	x		x	x	x	x	x
TX		x	x	x*			x	x	x	x	x	x	x	x	x
UT			x	x				x	x	x	x			x	x
VT			x		2			x	x	x	x	x			x
VA		x	x	x	123		x	x	x		x	x	x	x	x
WA	x		x	x	1234	x	x	x	x	x	x	x	x		x
WV	x	x	x	x	12	x	x	x	x	x	x		x	x	x
WI		x			2			x			x		x		x
WY			x			x	x	x	x	x	x	x	x	x	x

Table 7.4   (continued)

Key to Table 7.4

I.   Access to Care

    1. Open enrollment period

    2. No preexisting conditions exclusions

    3. Marketing restrictions

    4   Direct access to specific specialist

        X = obstetrician/gynecologist

        * = other (i.e., optometrist, dermatologist, chiropractor)

    5. Access to specific services

        1 = maternity stay guidelines

        2 = mammography/cytologic screening exams

        3 = experimental (i.e., bone marrow transplants for treatment
            of cancer)

        4 = mastectomy/reconstructive surgery

    6. Emergency care

    7. Any willing provider

II. Quality of Care

    8. Certificate of authority/license

    9. Medical audit/exam

    10. Quality requirements

III. Financing

    11. Financial requirements

    12. No gag rules/full disclosure of financial incentives

IV. Consumer Protection

    13. Evidence of coverage

    14. Confidentiality of medical information

    15. Complaint/grievance system

Note:

- IN: emergency care is provided for Medicaid recipient
- MI: direct access is provided for Medicaid recipient
- MA: confidentiality of medical information protects communications made to psychotherapists
- MT: any willing provider legislation is for dentists
- AL, LA, NH, NM, NC, ND, SD, TX: any willing provider legislation is for pharmacists
- VA: any willing provider legislation is for podiatrists

Although the major goal of "Any Willing Provider" legislation is to protect providers, such legislation is also an attempt to promote access to care. "Any Willing Provider" legislation compels managed care plans to enroll any provider who is willing to accept the plans' payment system, credentialing system, and quality standards (Avery 1995). Such legislation improves access to care because more providers may participate in managed care plans. By the end of 1997, 25 states had enacted legislation allowing providers to join a managed care plan if the provider met the terms of the plan. For example, South Carolina prohibits managed care plans from refusing any licensed physician, podiatrist, optometrist, or oral surgeon who wants to join from participating as a provider in the organization on the basis of his or her profession (S.C. Code Ann. 1996).

Only managed plans that meet certain requirements are allowed to provide care in the Medicaid program. States have also turned to credentialing to ensure that managed care plans provide Medicaid recipients access to appropriate medical care. Most states require that managed care plans provide access to services 24 hours per day. Some states require that providers see patients within certain time limits—24 hours for non-emergency urgent care and 4–6 weeks for routine care. States vary dramatically with respect to how precisely they specify access to specialty services. The Delaware contract with managed care plans, for example, argues "because there are so many factors involved in judging the adequacy of specialty provider networks, specification of a single standard ratio [of the number of specialists to the number of enrollees] is inappropriate . . . MCOs should clearly demonstrate that their proposed specialist network have sufficient capacity to service the planned number of DSHP clients [Medicaid beneficiaries in Delaware]; MCOs should show how they arrived at their network design by specifying the type and intensity of specialist services they expect to deliver to the enrolled population" (State of Delaware 1995). Florida, on the other hand, is more specific about the specialists that must be provided. Florida provides that "The Plan shall assure the availability of the following specialists, as appropriate for both adult and pediatric enrollees, on at least a referral basis, cardiologist, orthopedist, urologist, dermatologist, otolaryngologist, chiropractic physician, podiatrist, gastroenterologist, oncologist, radiologist, pathologist, anesthesiologist, psychiatrist, oral surgeon, physical therapist and a specialist in AIDS care (infectious disease specialist)" (Florida 1995).

Access implications for Medicare

As more Medicare beneficiaries with chronic illnesses enroll in managed care plans, the federal government should review the direct access laws passed by states. Direct access legislation allows individuals to choose a specialist as their primary care gatekeeper or to seek specialty care (providers or services) directly without using a primary care gatekeeper. Specialists may be the logical primary caregiver for some chronically ill Medicare beneficiaries. For example, an oncologist may be the primary caregiver for cancer patients. One possibility is to guarantee that a Medicare beneficiary could select his or her own primary caregiver (either a generalist or specialist). Medicare beneficiaries should be given this option.

Certain services, such as home health and durable medical equipment warrant special attention because chronically ill beneficiaries use them frequently (Table 7.2). The Medicare program should monitor access to these services in managed care plans to ensure that individuals have appropriate access. Access for chronically ill Medicare beneficiaries should be monitored extensively.

Regulating access to care is not costless. First, the access to care provisions interfere with the ability of the managed care plan to develop a delivery system and select a panel of providers that reflects the marketplace. Also, the provisions intrude upon the managed care plan's ability to develop a healthcare system that mirrors their own perception of the enrollees' needs. The managed care plan, for example, may develop an alternative to home health care. From the perspective of risk adjustment, however, the main advantage is that the access to care provisions prevent certain managed care plans from selecting providers or services that will not appeal to the chronically ill. By carefully tailoring the regulations to monitor services used disproportionately by the chronically ill, especially for services where there have been reports of inadequate care, the Medicare program could increase the likelihood that all managed care plans would be appropriate for the chronically ill. This would reduce the level of risk selection for chronically ill Medicare beneficiaries in managed care plans.

Quality of Care

States have enacted several different types of legislation designed to monitor and improve the quality of care provided by managed care plans. At a minimum, managed care plans are typically required to obtain a license or certificate of need to operate in a specific state. The state insurance commissioner usually oversees the licensing process, monitors fiscal solvency requirements, and oversees marketing practices. Most states require managed care plans to collect uniform data, conduct medical audits, and become accredited.

Presently 47 states plus the District of Columbia require some form of medical audit, typically occurring every three years. These audits often include evaluations of quality assurance, utilization review, peer review, patient-grievance procedures, as well as patient-satisfaction issues such as wait times for appointments and specialist referral rules. Medical audits may examine all aspects of a plan's performance or focus on specific indicators of plan performance. Much of the legislation governing medical audits is quite general. For example, the District of Columbia conducts a universal medical audit that provides a single overall assessment of the performance of managed care plans (DC Code 1997). Maryland uses a more targeted approach analyzing specific aspects of managed care plans' performance before aggregating the data to reach an overall opinion (MD Health General Code 1997). Specific aspects included in Maryland reviews are whether baseline clinical examinations are conducted, complaints of enrollees, an enrollee satisfaction survey and other quality of care indicators. Maine, Wyoming, and the District of Columbia all require managed care plans to establish and maintain procedures ensuring that the healthcare services provided to enrollees are of reasonable quality with professionally recognized standards of medical practice (MRS 1996; Wyo. Stat. 1997; DC Code 1997).

State Medicaid programs employ a variety of approaches for credentialing health plans to make sure they meet minimally acceptable standards. Many states have relied on private accreditation bodies to monitor quality of care. Some states impose higher standards for managed care plans that want to enroll chronically ill Medicaid beneficiaries such as the SSI population. By imposing strict credentialing requirements, the Medicare programs could assure that all managed care plans meet high standards.

In 1996, 23 states contracted with any plan that met the state's qualifications and the price the state was willing to pay. Twelve states contracted with selected plans using a competitive process in 1996 (Rosenbaum et al. 1997). The competitive process always contains a set of plan qualifications that must be met and may include price as one of the relevant factors. Until recently states have focused their attention on the healthcare needs of a relatively healthy young family population. They are only beginning to address the specific capabilities that plans will need in order to serve high need subpopulations (e.g., disabled children or adults, persons with HIV/AIDS, or elderly persons) (Rosenbaum et al. 1997).

The Arizona AHCCCS program provides an example of how a Medicaid program has incorporated aspect of quality in its credentialing process. Arizona evaluates programs in several broad categories: personnel qualifications, program standards, organizational structure, and the plan's network. Each component is then scored and plans are allowed to participate based on their score and their cost. The number of health plans that meet the qualification standards varies from locality to locality, but statewide more than half are denied contracts because they do not meet credentialing requirements or because their bid was too high (McCall 1996). In 1995, for example, AHCCCS awarded contracts to 39 out of 95 bidders.

A number of Medicaid programs have used a similar process to restrict the number of plans that can enroll Medicaid beneficiaries, and in some cases the state has given a monopoly to a single managed care plan. The District of Columbia, for example, has given an exclusive franchise to a single managed care plan to provide services to all children with SSI eligibility (HCFA 1996). New Jersey requires all Medicaid beneficiaries with mental disabilities and addictions in a geographic area to enroll in a single managed care group. In order for a managed care plan to qualify to provide services to this group it must have: (1) at least three years' experience providing publicly supported mental health and substance abuse services; (2) experience in risk contracting for mental health services; and (3) experience with populations with other special healthcare needs, including experience with enrollees from linguistic and cultural minorities, children and adults with AIDS, and children receiving child protective services.

In addition to state licensure, some large employers have recently demanded that managed care organizations meet additional standards established by private accrediting bodies such as the National Committee for Quality Assurance (NCQA). The accreditation standards are often similar to licensure requirements but may exceed the licensing standards established by states.

These are a good beginning but do not begin to address the wide range of chronic illnesses in the Medicare population. For many chronic illnesses no quality measures have been developed. Given the high percentage of Medicare expenditures devoted to the care of the chronically ill, clearly more attention needs to be given to developing quality of care measures for this population. Incorporation of additional measures for chronically ill Medicare beneficiaries will help ensure a minimum level of care provided to the chronically ill. As a result, less risk selection will occur because Medicare beneficiaries may assume that all managed care plans are maintaining a high minimum quality standard.

Quality of care implications for Medicare

Many Medicaid programs and private sector employers have created a two-tiered accreditation (credentialing) process—plans that meet only the minimum standards established by the state and plans that meet the state's standards plus the higher standards of the accreditation (credentialing) body. HCFA should consider this approach when creating credential requirements for managed care plans for the chronically ill. Such plans would be more comprehensive by meeting private accreditation (and credentialing) standards in addition to state licensing requirements.

The Medicare program has two options. The first option is to insist that all managed care plans meet a standard of care beyond current requirements. The standard of care should be appropriate care for the chronically ill Medicare beneficiary. The second option is to create two levels of accreditation and for Medicare to pay a higher rate to plans that meet this higher level of accreditation. There are precedents for a two-tiered process of accreditation and licensure in other areas of healthcare. Hospitals, for example, are not permitted to receive federal funding for residency programs unless the hospitals meet both the federal standards and the private standards established by the Joint Commission on Accreditation of Healthcare Organizations (JCAHO). Direct and indirect medical education payments under Medicare's prospective payment system are dependent on the hospital's receiving JCAHO accreditation.

Having higher accreditation or credentialing requirements necessitates the development of better quality of care measures specifically designed for the chronically ill. HEDIS 3.0, the latest version of quality measures developed by the NCQA, contains only two measures that are designed to measure the quality of care for the chronically ill. The two measures are: (1) appropriate medications for people with asthma; and (2) eye examinations for people with diabetes. In addition, some measures are being evaluated for inclusion in a future reporting set, including monitoring the diabetic patient's blood level, prevention of stroke in patients with atrial fibrillation, ensuring that individuals with congestive heart failure receive appropriate outpatient care, management of cholesterol for patients with coronary artery disease, controlling high blood pressure in people with hypertension, assessing the appropriateness of treatment for breast cancer patients, and assessing the appropriateness of prescription drugs for individuals with HIV-related pneumonia.

Financing

To become licensed, a managed care plan will usually need to demonstrate financial responsibility. Typically the state commissioner grants a managed care plan a certificate of authority after the plan presents data to demonstrate financial responsibility, adequate working capital, or other financial requirements. Most states impose financial requirements to ensure that managed care plans will remain financially stable and able to provide services to their enrollees. Plans may be required to show financial statements including assets, liabilities, sources of financial support, and financial feasibility plans (MCL 1997).

At the end of 1997, 46 states plus the District of Columbia had enacted legislation governing the financial responsibilities of managed care plans, including capitalization and reserve requirements. These are basically savings required for both initial purposes and for future protection against insolvency.

States are becoming increasingly concerned about the financial incentives for physicians paid on either a fully-capitated or partially-capitated basis and whether patients are aware of the financial incentives that apply to their personal physicians. States are also concerned that health plan members can obtain information about the financial incentives faced by their individual physicians. Many states have banned "gag rules" that prohibit physicians from discussing certain treatment alternatives with their patients. By late 1997, 24 states and the District of Columbia had enacted legislation prohibiting managed care contracts from containing gag rules. The specific language of anti-gag rules varies from state to state, though it typically prohibits a contract provision from forbidding a healthcare provider from communicating certain information necessary for the delivery of healthcare services to a health plan member. For example, the District of Columbia law states that "no contract between a health maintenance organization and provider shall prohibit, impede, or interfere in the discussion between a patient and a provider of medical treatment option including discussion regarding financial coverage of those treatment options" (DC 1997). The District of Columbia law further states that "a contract between a carrier and provider shall permit and require the provider to discuss medical treatment options with the patient" (DC 1997).

Some managed care plans have attempted to keep financial arrangements with their providers confidential. A few states, however, are requiring managed care plans to make these arrangements publicly available. Public disclosure helps consumers make informed decisions by comparing health plans. Also, public disclosure forces managed care plans to be honest and open about their coverage to enrollees and potential enrollees. New Jersey, for example, requires that managed care plans give the Health Department copies of their contract agreements (NJ Stat. 1996).

Financing implications for Medicare

The recent regulations promulgated by Medicare address some of these issues. The new regulations permit physician groups to be at risk without stop loss insurance if they have at least 25,000 individuals in their risk panels. The individuals can be insured by Medicare, Medicaid, or commercial insurers. If managed care plans have fewer than 25,000 enrollees, the managed care plan is required to purchase individual stop loss insurance.

The current Medicare regulations do very little to protect the managed care plan, the physician group, or the individual physician who is at risk and has a high percentage of chronically ill individuals. Individual stop loss insurance does not protect the physician against a panel of patients whose health status is below the Medicare average. Even if the Medicare beneficiary exceeds the dollar threshold and triggers the reinsurance, the managed care plan, physician group, or individual physician will "lose money" on that particular patient because of the difference between the payment and the stop loss threshold. In other words, the most recent Medicare regulations do little to protect the chronically ill Medicare beneficiary or the provider who happens to enroll that individual. As a result, the recent regulations will do little to reduce the level of risk selection.

The Medicare program should carefully review the financial requirements imposed by the states. Special attention should be given to the amount of risk a physician or physician group can accept. Special attention should also be given to prohibiting gag rules by any managed care plan participating in the Medicare program.

Consumer Protection

States are enacting various laws to protect the consumer. Many observers suggest that these consumer protection laws may promote quality and restore consumer trust in the healthcare system (Aston 1997). Consumer protections may include disclosing information to healthcare plan enrollees and potential enrollees and ensuring confidentiality of patient information. An important consumer protection is whether health plan members are provided the information necessary to allow them to purchase policies with full information and then ensuring that managed care plans fulfill their policies (Iglehart 1997).

Most states require managed care organizations to provide evidence of coverage, information about material changes in coverage, a list of available health services, a description of how to resolve enrollees' complaints, and an annual statement of their financial condition to their enrollees. Currently, 41 states plus the District of Columbia require managed care organizations to take specific steps to guarantee the confidentiality of their medical information. Rhode Island, for example, prohibits managed care plans from sending enrollee-specific information (which is not essential for the compilation of statistical data related to enrollees) to any international, national, regional, or local medical information data base (RI Gen. Laws 1996).

Some consumer protection regulations require managed care plans to develop due process procedures that safeguard the consumer's rights. By requiring managed care plans to establish systems for receiving and resolving grievances, consumers are assured that their rights and interests are being protected. When managed care plans deny treatment or services, due process procedures may be useful to guarantee the disclosure of information and compliance with the complaint process. Florida, for example, created a statewide managed care ombudsman committee (FL Stat. 1996). The ombudsman committee receives complaints regarding quality of care in managed care plans and assists the state agency with regulatory authority over managed care to investigate and resolve the complaints. New Jersey has enacted legislation that allows patients to pursue a non-binding appeal with an independent utilization review body in grievance actions involving utilization review decisions (NJSN 1996). California (31), Missouri (32), and Texas (33) have installed toll-free numbers for consumer complaints about managed care plans (Cal. Wel. and Inst. Code 1996; Mo. 1997; Tex. Inst. Code 1997). Maryland requires managed care plans to provide "24 hour access by telephone to a person who is able to appropriately respond to calls from members and providers concerning after-hours care" and a 24-hour toll-free number for use in hospital emergency departments (MD Health-General Code Ann. 1997). Additionally, Arizona, California, Connecticut, New Jersey, and Rhode Island have all enacted some form of external appeals legislation for managed care grievances.

Consumer protection implications for Medicare

HCFA should adopt a combination of the state approaches on information disclosure. It should be possible to suspend participation in the Medicare program of plans that receive a large number of complaints. This would reduce the incentive to under-treat the chronically ill to achieve favorable risk selection.

RECOMMENDATIONS FOR MEDICARE

Based on an analysis of Medicare data on the cost of services for chronically ill Medicare beneficiaries and the services they utilize, state regulatory and credentialing requirements, and HCFA's current policies, the following recommendations are presented:

1. *HCFA should focus its regulatory and credentialing efforts on problems of access for the chronically ill Medicare beneficiaries.* Managed care plans have a strong financial incentive to discourage the enrollment of chronically ill individuals in the absence of adequate risk adjusters.

2. *HCFA should focus on access to specific services.* The chronically ill are much more likely to use certain services than the "typical" Medicare beneficiary. Services that are heavily utilized by chronically ill Medicare beneficiaries include durable medical equipment,

home health agencies, and certain physician specialties. HCFA should focus its surveillance efforts on these services because they are likely to be the services managed care plans will utilize to discourage the enrollment of the chronically ill. An ombudsman would help to monitor chronically ill individuals' access to specific services.

3. *HCFA should make sure that the chronically ill have access to appropriate providers.* States have developed a variety of laws to ensure that the chronically ill have access to appropriate providers including access to all participating health plans, direct access to certain providers, and access to specific services. HCFA should review these state laws and incorporate the best provisions into Medicare regulations. This could prevent managed care plans from developing a set of providers that is unattractive to the chronically ill.

4. *HCFA should make sure that the financial arrangements that managed care plans have with their physicians encourage physicians to enroll the chronically ill.* In the absence of risk adjusters, capitated physicians who treat a disproportionate share of chronically ill individuals will be at a serious financial disadvantage. The most recent HCFA regulations do little to address this issue. HCFA should determine if the financial incentives created by its own payment system or by the managed care plans create financial incentives that penalize physicians who specialize in the care of the chronically ill. HCFA should severely restrict health plans from placing individual physicians at financial risk unless the managed care plan has incorporated adequate risk adjusters into the payment system for individual physicians.

5. *HCFA should require managed care plans to pay capitated physicians more to care for the chronically ill.* This would ensure that physicians with a specialty that attracts the chronically ill will not suffer financially and will not withhold necessary and appropriate care to the chronically ill.

6. *HCFA should develop standards that ensure that all managed care plans are able to provide care for the chronically ill. Alternatively, HCFA should establish a higher standard of care and only managed care plans meeting this standard would be recommended for the chronically ill.* Some states have imposed stricter criteria for health plans that want to provide care to Supplemental Security Income (SSI) beneficiaries. Medicare should adopt these more comprehensive credentialing requirements for the Medicare population. HEDIS and other accreditation tools should place greater emphasis on developing measures that apply to the chronically ill.

7. *HCFA should require managed care plans to report uniform data.* Many states require health plans to provide information on benefits,

service network, grievance procedures, and other pertinent information in a uniform manner. This would allow Medicare beneficiaries to do more comparison shopping and would minimize the effects of marketing that lead to risk selection. Much more attention should be given to data on the chronically ill, which represent a very large proportion of Medicare spending.

8. *HCFA should create an ombudsman to monitor the quality of care and to catalog beneficiary complaints.* HCFA needs to create an information system that monitors consumer complaints and catalogs them in a coherent format. It would serve as an early warning system for the Administrator.

THE BALANCED BUDGET ACT

The Balanced Budget Act (BBA) of 1997 included significant changes in the Medicare program. One change that is particularly relevant to the issue of plan regulation is the expansion in private plan options for beneficiaries (e.g, medical savings accounts, provider-sponsored organizations, and private indemnity plans), especially given the new provisions restricting disenrollment that are described in Chapter 8 (Moon, Gage, and Evans 1997). Concerns have been raised that some of the new private plan options are subject to less consumer protection and oversight than Medicare's current private plan options. For example, the Secretary of Health and Human Services has little authority to control premium growth or establish a standard benefit package. Fewer consumer protections/oversight of some plans combined with changes in enrollment and disenrollment rules that require beneficiaries to choose or switch plans during the one-month open enrollment period (or during their first three months in a new plan) could negatively affect chronically ill Medicare beneficiaries. For example, if chronically ill Medicare beneficiaries choose a health plan during open enrollment but discover that the plan does not adequately meet their needs (e.g., limited access to specialty care), they may have to wait until next year's open enrollment period to change plans. This is also a problem if they develop a medical condition after open enrollment and their needs change. With restricted freedom to leave plans at any time, a greater degree of regulation, credentialing, and monitoring of quality and appropriate standards of care becomes even more important.

REFERENCES

Anderson, G., E. Steinberg, J. Whittle, N. Powe, S. Antebi, and R. Herbert. 1990. "Development of Clinical and Economic Prognoses from Medicare Claims Data." *Journal of the American Medical Association* 263 (7): 967–72.

Aston, G. 1997. "Discord on Managed Care Standards." *American Medical News* 40 (1): 74–75.

Avery, L. P. 1995. "Debate about 'Any Willing Provider' Laws Continues in 1995." *AORN Journal* 61 (3): 597–98.

Azevedo, D. 1996. "Will the States Get Tough with HMOs? Anti-Managed Care Proposals Pile Up Nationwide." *Medical Economics* 73 (16): 172–85.

Bodenheimer, T. 1996. "The HMO Backlash—Righteous or Reactionary?" *New England Journal of Medicine* 335: 1601–4.

Health Care Financing Administration (HCFA). 1996. *Medicaid Managed Care Report, 1996.* Washington, DC.

Hoffman, C., D. Rice, and H. Sung. 1996. "Persons with Chronic Conditions." *Journal of the American Medical Association* 276 (18): 1473–79.

Iglehart, J. K. 1997. "State Regulation of Managed Care: NAIC President Josephine Musser." *Health Affairs* 16 (6): 36–39.

Ireys, H. T., G. F. Anderson, T. J. Shaffer, and J. M. Neff. 1997. "Expenditures for Care of Children with Chronic Illnesses Enrolled in the Washington State Medicaid Program, Fiscal Year 1993." *Pediatrics* 100 (2): 197–204.

McCall, N. 1996. "The Arizona Health Care Cost Containment System: Thirteen Years of Managed Care in Medicaid." The Henry J. Kaiser Family Foundation.

Moon, M., B. Gage, and A. Evans. 1997. *An Examination of Key Medicare Provisions in the Balanced Budget Act of 1997.* Report to the Commonwealth Fund.

Neff, J. M., and G. F. Anderson. 1995. "Protecting Children with Chronic Illness in a Competitive Marketplace." *Journal of the American Medical Association* 274 (23): 1866–69.

Rosenbaum, S., P. Shin, B. Smith, E. Wehr, P. Borzi, M. Zakheim, K. Shaw, and K. Silver. 1997. "Negotiating the New Health System: A Nationwide Study of Medicaid Managed Care Contracts." Washington, DC: The George Washington University Medical Center, Center for Health Policy Research.

State of Delaware Department of Health and Human Services Request for Proposal for MCOs, II.51, 1995.

Statutes:

Ark. Stat. Ann. @ 23-99-303 (1995)

Cal. Wel. & Inst. Code @ 1368.02 (1996)

D.C. Code @ 25-4506 (1997)

16 Del. C. @ 9106 (1996)

Florida's Medicaid Prepaid Health Plans, 1995

FL Stat. @ 641.60 (1996)

KRS @ 304.17A-171 (1996)

MCL @ 333.21021 (1997)

MD Health-General Code Ann. @ 19-705.1 (1997)

Mo. HB 335 (1997)

M.R.S. 24-A @4204 (1996)

N.C. Gen. Stat. @ 58-51-45 (1996)

NJ Stat. @ 641.60 (1996)
NJSN 269 (1996)
O.C.G.A. @ 33-24-56 (1995)
RI Gen. Laws @ 5-37. 3-4 (1996)
S.C. Code Ann. @ 38-33-290 (1996)
Tex. Inst. Code art. 21.72 (1997)
Wyo. Stat. @ 26-34-108 (1997)

8

Monitoring Disenrollment from HMOs[1]

Joy de Beyer

T he strategies discussed in earlier chapters—coordinated open enrollment, provision of unbiased and timely information to beneficiaries, better oversight of marketing, partial standardization of benefit packages, and more stringent oversight and credentialing of plans— will primarily affect beneficiary decisions at the time of enrollment. After beneficiaries have enrolled, it is easy for an HMO to determine which members are using more resources than provided for in the capitated premium. With a bit of additional analysis and judgment, the plan can make reasonably good estimates of which enrollees are likely to continue to use more resources in the coming year than are provided for in the capitation. Although it is not easy for plans or providers to act on this information without fear of violating either professional ethics or public trust, the financial incentives to do so are so great that it would be worthwhile for HCFA to raise the cost of encouraging selective disenrollment.

This chapter takes stock of what we know about disenrollment from Medicare HMOs. It examines rates, trends and reasons, and the effect of disenrollment on risk selection. It asks whether there is any evidence that plans are encouraging high-risk enrollees to disenroll and describes HCFA's oversight of disenrollment. At present, Medicare beneficiaries can disenroll from their HMO at any time and for any reason, and disenrollment becomes effective at the end of the month. The BBA changes this, moving toward a system by 2002 where disenrollment is allowed only in November, except under circumstances that are detailed later in the chapter. The chapter considers how the new restrictions on disenrollment in the BBA may affect the picture, and whether financial penalties should be imposed on HMOs with unusually high (or selective) disenrollment.

Disenrollment is of concern for two main reasons. First, if disenrollees are especially in need of care and are exiting plans because they have received poor care, this highlights concerns about the quality of care provided for the sickest beneficiaries under managed care. Second, if disenrollees who return to fee-for-service are disproportionately those with above average needs for care and are thus more expensive than the average beneficiary, Medicare expenditures will rise. If high-cost enrollees are leaving certain plans and switching to others, the receiving plans are at financial risk, which is also a problem.

Even if disenrollment rates are low, the financial impact of selective disenrollment can be substantial. Medical expenditures are so skewed that even a small number of high-cost disenrollees can have a significant effect on HMOs' bottom lines and on Medicare outlays. For example, if disenrollees have 42 percent higher expenditures than continuous enrollees and disenrollees account for as little as 3 percent of total enrollment, then selective disenrollment would improve the HMO case mix, relative to the capitation payments, by approximately 1.5 percent per year.[2] Other things equal, selective disenrollment of this magnitude would increase HMO profits by 1.5 percent of premiums per year. Over a period of a few years, even this very low level of disenrollment would clearly be a significant contributor to risk selection.

Of course, not all disenrollment is profitable to plans. Marketing costs for recruiting new enrollees are substantial, and disenrollment represents a loss of the marketing and administrative costs associated with those enrollees and reduces plan revenues. Moreover, fixed overhead costs are substantial and contribute to the need for a large enrollee base for profitable and efficient management of a plan. Thus, plans have an interest in reducing disenrollment, except for beneficiaries whose healthcare costs are persistently higher than their Medicare capitation rate.

DISENROLLMENT RATES AND TRENDS

Disenrollment rates have fallen since the risk program began, as reflected in Table 8.1.[3] Disenrollment was very high early in the Medicare risk demonstrations: on average, 23 percent of all those who enrolled during 1984 disenrolled within 12 months (Brown et al. 1986). Disenrollment rates were much higher (7 percent to 27 percent) in multiple plan markets than in single

Table 8.1 Study Findings of National Disenrollment Rates for Medicare HMOs

Study	Year/s Studied	Data Source	Disenrollment Findings
Brown et al. (1986)	Enrollees in 1984	17 HMOs in ten market areas participating in Medicare compet-ition demonstration	Percent who disenrolled within 12 months of enrolling was 23% average, 6.6%–27% in markets with multiple HMOs, 4.4%–6.3% in markets with a single plan
Langwell et al. (1993)	1985–1988	109 risk plans with total enrollment of more than 830,000	20% disenrolled within 12 months and 33% within two years of enrolling
Riley, Ingber, and Tudor (1997)	1993, 1994, and 1995	HCFA enrollment database	1993 and 1994 annual rates (computed from monthly rates) of 11% and 14.2% (including people who moved out of the plan area of service, estimated at around 15% of all disenrollees)
Nelson et al. (1996)	1995	HCFA Group Health Plan (GHP) of all Medicare beneficiaries who enrolled in an HMO for at least two months between 3/1/95 and 3/1/96	Percent of Medicare benefici-aries who had disenrolled from a plan during retrospective 12-month period (1995), with at least two months enrollment; voluntary disenrollment of 7.5%
Dallek and Swirsky (1997)	1995, 1996, and first quarter of 1997	HCFA monthly disenrollment data, all HMOs with average Medicare enrollment greater than 1,000 and at least 12 months' participation	Sum of monthly disenrollment, as percentage of average annual enrollment. Recent rising trend, from 11% in 1995, 13% in 1996, and 17% in 1997, if first four months are representative of rest of the year

plan markets, where rates ranged between 4 and 6 percent. Subsequent studies found progressively lower disenrollment rates. Twenty percent of the 830,000 beneficiaries who enrolled in HMOs between 1985 and 1988 disenrolled within 12 months of enrolling (Langwell et al. 1993). Of a sample of new enrollees in 1993, 16 percent had disenrolled after 12 months (Riley, Ingber, and Tudor 1997).[4] After about a decade of managed care in Medicare, disenrollment rates are down significantly.

Methodological differences in the way that disenrollment rates are defined and calculated make comparisons across studies hazardous and make it very hard to assess recent trends. Riley, Ingber, and Tudor (1997) calculate annualized disenrollment rates of 11 percent in 1993 and 14 percent in 1994, using HCFA monthly disenrollment data.[5] Dallek and Swirsky (1997) used the same data to compute 1995 and 1996 average Medicare HMO annual disenrollment rates of 11 percent and 13 percent respectively for plans that had participated in Medicare for at least a year and had an average membership of at least 1,000.[6] Only 7.5 percent of 3.3 million Medicare beneficiaries who had been enrolled in a risk HMO for at least two months during the year ending February 1996 or were enrolled in a plan on March 1, 1996 had disenrolled from a plan during the 12 months March 1995–February 1996 (Nelson et al. 1996).[7] The exclusion of people who had been enrolled for less than two months during the year biases this measure of disenrollment downward quite substantially: people who disenrolled before enrollment became final or within the first three months of enrollment accounted for more than one in four (28.0 percent) disenrollees during 1996.

Dallek and Swirsky note that disenrollment rates have risen since 1995 from 11 percent to 13 percent in 1996, and appear, on the basis of the first quarter of 1997, to have risen further. However, they caution that the 1997 data are preliminary and subject to change after being audited and "cleaned." Without additional research and analysis, it is not possible to judge whether these data should raise a red flag for policymakers' attention. Disenrollment rates are very strongly related to the length of time plans have been contracting with Medicare and the size of their Medicare membership—plans with large numbers of Medicare enrollees that also tend to have been contracting with Medicare for longer periods of time have lower disenrollment rates than plans with fewer Medicare enrollees and whose Medicare participation is more recent (Dallek and Swirsky 1997). Markets with more HMOs tend to have more disenrollment because people switch among competing HMOs. So if, in fact, disenrollment rates have been rising recently, this may be because consumers are taking advantage of choice and competition as new plans enter the market, and it may reflect the inexperience of newly participating HMOs. The latter should be transitional; the former is the result of well functioning markets. Clearly, disenrollment rates need to be watched and studied further and a standard methodology agreed upon for calculating annual rates.

REASONS FOR DISENROLLMENT

People disenroll for many different reasons, only some of which raise concerns about quality of care, fair play, and fair payment. Disenrollment may be involuntary or voluntary. Involuntary disenrollment occurs because beneficiaries die; they move out of the plan service area; they lose their Medicare Part B eligibility; employers or former employers drop the plan from their benefit package; or plans drop out of the risk program. A 1996 survey of 990 disenrollees found that about 20 percent of disenrollment was involuntary (Nelson et al. 1996). Voluntary disenrollment is in response to factors that "push" beneficiaries out of a plan: dissatisfaction with its providers or operating rules, dissatisfaction with access to care (especially referrals to specialists), inconvenience of care location, or an increase in the premium or reduction in benefits. Voluntary disenrollment is also in response to "pull" factors: enrollees decide that another plan is more attractive, given a comparison of relative costs and benefits. Of those who voluntarily leave their plans, about 40 percent opt for fee-for-service and 60 percent switch to another plan. Among beneficiaries who switch to another HMO, many are drawn by a better deal, but the percentage who are motivated by dissatisfaction with plan physicians is about the same as among disenrollees to fee-for-service (see Table 8.2). Overall, many more of the moves into fee-for-service are motivated by dissatisfaction with a plan, especially being denied access to care, and misunderstandings of HMO rules.[8]

EVIDENCE THAT DISENROLLMENT IS SELECTIVE

This section summarizes the evidence showing that disenrollees are on average sicker than those who remain enrolled, using the same three indicators as for measuring risk selection of managed care enrollees—health status, use of services, and mortality. Where the research findings permit, data on disenrollees to fee-for-service are reported separately from those on beneficiaries who switched to other plans.

Health Status

Medicare beneficiaries who disenroll from HMOs and return to fee-for-service generally have poorer health status than their counterparts who remain enrolled. This was the case in the early years of Medicare managed care and remains so today; no contrary findings have been published. Surveys found that people who disenrolled within 12 months of enrolling during 1984 were more likely than other plan members to report their health status as poor at the time of enrollment, less likely to be able to perform instrumental activities of daily living, and more likely to have a health problem possibly requiring hospitalization (Brown et al. 1986; Tucker and Langwell 1989). They also tended to be older and poorer, correlates of higher risk. Ten years later, sicker people are still more likely to disenroll to go back to fee-for-service than healthier HMO enrollees. The GAO analyzed

Table 8.2 Reasons for Disenrolling from Medicare Risk Plans

Percent Citing the Most Important Reason as:	All Who Disenrolled	Disenrollees to Fee-for-Service	Switchers from One Plan to Another
Involuntary disenrollment (predominantly because individual moved out of plan service area)	19.8%	28.1	14.9%*
Location inconvenient or beneficiary moved too far from plan doctors	8.6	4.2	11.2*
Physician left plan, died, or retired	6.6	1.2	9.7*
"Pulled" by more attractive option			
Another plan costs less	1.8	1.1	2.2
Another plan offers better benefits	12.4	8.5	14.7*
Reached limits on prescription coverage	1.5	0.4	2.2
Factors indicating dissatisfaction			
Dissatisfied with plan physicians	24.4	25.1	24.2
Plan too expensive	7.8	7.7	7.8
Access problems—could not get specialist referrals, a appointments, home health, or admission to hospital when needed	6.4	10.0	4.3*
Misunderstanding of HMO rules	2.0	4.4	0.5*
Other (including: friend, relative, or doctor recommended change; not treated as an individual; bills not paid; became sicker as a plan member)	8.6	9.4	8.2
Total	100	100	100
Number	990	559	431

*Difference between switchers and disenrollees to fee-for-service is statistically significant at the .01 level, two-tailed test.

Source: Nelson, L., et al. 1996. *Access to Care in Medicare Managed Care: Results from a 1996 Survey of Enrollees and Disenrollees.* Washington, DC: Physician Payment Review Commission, 57.

data on California beneficiaries who enrolled in an HMO in 1994 or 1995, comparing those who disenrolled within six months with those who remained enrolled, with respect to five chronic conditions (USGAO/HEHS 1997).[9] Six percent of all new enrollees returned to fee-for-service within six months, but this rate varied greatly depending on whether beneficiaries had one or more of the five chronic conditions: only 4.5 percent of those with none of the five chronic conditions, 6.7 percent of those with one, and 10.2 percent of those with two or more conditions disenrolled to fee-for-service within six months. The pattern persisted when the sample was disaggregated by age, as shown in Table 8.3 below.

The 1996 beneficiary survey analyzed by Nelson et al. found disenrollees to fee-for-service to be in poorer health and more likely to have functional impairments than continuous enrollees or those who had switched from one HMO to another. (In the quotation that follows, "current enrollees" denotes continuous enrollees and people who switched from one HMO to another, and disenrollees refers only to people who disenrolled from an HMO into fee-for-service.)

> For example, 14 percent of disenrollees reported they were in poor health and 13 percent reported needing assistance with bathing, compared with 4 percent and 6 percent, respectively, for current enrollees. Disenrollees were more likely to be the non-elderly disabled, the oldest old, African American, have low incomes, and be dually covered by Medicaid, all groups that tend to be higher risk. In addition, among the elderly, disenrollees were more likely to have been entitled to Medicare due to disability before reaching the age of 65. Disenrollees were remarkably similar to current enrollees in the proportion with specific medical conditions such as diabetes, cancer, heart disease and arthritis (with the exception of strokes). However, a higher percentage of disenrollees had four or more of these conditions. Disenrollees worried more about their health and were twice as likely to visit their doctors more than once per month. (Nelson et al. 1996, 38).

Table 8.3 Disenrollment to Fee-for-Service Within Six Months of Enrollment, 1993 and 1994, for All California Medicare HMO Enrollees, by Chronic Condition and Age

	All New Enrollees	65–69	70–74	75–84	85+
All	6.0	4.6	5.6	7.0	8.3
No Chronic Conditions	4.5	3.4	4.2	5.7	6.5
1 Chronic Condition	6.7	6.1	6.5	6.9	8.4
2 or More Chronic Conditions	10.2	8.9	10.0	10.6	11.6

Source: United States General Accounting Office. 1997. *Medicare: Fewer and Lower Cost Beneficiaries with Chronic Conditions Enroll in HMOs.* Report to the Chairman, Subcommittee of Health, Committee on Ways and Means, House of Representatives. GAO/HEHS-97-160. Washington, DC: Table 5.

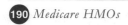

Table 8.4   Comparison Between Medicare Risk HMO Enrollees
and Disenrollees

	Current Medicare Risk Enrollees (includes switchers)	Disenrollees to Fee-for Service
Demographic and Socioeconomic Characteristics		
Age		
< 65 (disabled)	5.4	9.4*
> 85	7.6	11.5
Race		
African-American	7.7	13.1*
Percent Medicaid buy-in	3.8	11.5[†]
Percent of enrollees aged 65 and over who were originally entitled to Medicare as a result of disability	6.2	10.2[‡]
Income		
< $10,000	19.9	27.8*
Education		
8 years or less	14.1	18.4[§]
Mean number of months enrolled in plan	35.5	23.7[†]

Continued

Table 8.4 reproduces results from this survey showing health status differences between current enrollees (including switchers) and those who had
disenrolled in favor of fee-for-service.

Mortality

Riley, Lubitz, and Rabey (1991) compared mortality rates in 1987 for about
800,000 people who were enrolled in HMOs and more than 80,000 who
disenrolled from 108 Medicare HMOs. They used death rates for 13 million
Medicare beneficiaries in fee-for-service residing in the areas served by the
HMOs as a baseline. They computed "adjusted mortality ratios" (AMR),
actual deaths among the enrollee and disenrollee groups, as a ratio of the
death rates among fee-for-service beneficiaries, adjusted for age, sex, and
county of residence. The AMR for disenrollees was 1.23 ($p < .01$) and for
enrollees it was 0.80 ($p < .001$). Thus, disenrollees had much higher death
rates than enrollees or beneficiaries in fee-for-service, and enrollees had
lower death rates than beneficiaries in fee-for-service. All differences were
statistically significant. A study using more recent data found similar results: among nearly 17,000 people who disenrolled from HMOs in January
1994, 3.5 percent of those who reenrolled into another HMO died in 1994,
compared with 6.0 percent of those who disenrolled to fee-for-service (Riley
et al. 1997).[10]

Table 8.4   (continued)

	Current Medicare Risk Enrollees (includes switchers)	Disenrollees to Fee-for Service
Health and Functional Status		
Health Status		
Excellent	25.6	21.3*
Very good	31.8	24.6
Good	27.5	28.0
Fair	10.8	13.2
Poor	4.3	12.8
Percent with a history of selected conditions#		
Two conditions	25.5	20.6‡
Three	16.3	16.0
Four or more	18.8	23.5‡
Percent needing help with:		
Bathing	6.4	13.3†
Taking medicine	5.6	16.1†
Getting in and out of bed	2.6	5.9†
Travel	5.7	13.3†

Notes: #The conditions are: arteriosclerosis, hypertension, diabetes, myocardial infarction, angina, congestive heart failure, other heart condition, skin cancer, other types of cancer, stroke, rheumatoid arthritis, other arthritis, COPD, and asthma, emphysema, or other lung conditions. The only significant difference for percentages with any individual condition are for stroke, where 13.7 percent of disenrollees compared to only 8.1 percent of enrollees have a history of stroke.

  * Difference between current enrollees and disenrollees to fee-for-service in their distribution across categories is statistically significant at the .01 level, chi-square test.

  †Difference between current enrollees and disenrollees to fee-for-service is statistically significant at the .01 level, two-tailed test.

  ‡Difference between current enrollees and disenrollees to fee-for-service is statistically significant at the .05 level, two-tailed test.

  §Difference between current enrollees and disenrollees to fee-for-service in their distribution across categories is statistically significant at the .05 level, chi-square test.

  Source: Nelson, L., et al. 1996. *Access to Care in Medicare Managed Care: Results from a 1996 Survey of Enrollees and Disenrollees*. Washington, DC: Physician Payment Review Commission, 39–41.

The only other published study we found of comparative mortality rates among disenrollees was narrower in scope and showed variation among HMOs (Riley, Rabey, and Kasper 1989). It examined relative mortality risk for enrollees and disenrollees in three Medicare HMOs and comparable fee-for-service Medicare beneficiaries between 1980 and 1986. One of the HMOs clearly had favorable selection with respect to disenrollment, with relative mortality risk significantly higher (1.71, P = 0.003) for disenrollees during the two years after disenrollment compared to continuous enrollees. It was also higher than fee-for-service beneficiaries in the area (RR = 1.17). At the second HMO, disenrollees had a higher relative risk of death than enrollees (1.43), but this was not significantly different from the enrollees at the 5 percent level of significance (P = 0.101), possibly because of small sample size (n = 244), and was only marginally higher than fee-for-service beneficiaries in the area (RR = 1.05). The third HMO showed neutral disenrollment, with very similar relative risks of dying for disenrollees and enrollees (RR = 1.09) and the Medicare fee-for-service population in the area (RR = 1.01). A hypothetical mortality-based adjustment to the AAPCC would have reduced payments by 13 percent and 5 percent for the first two HMOs in the first year after enrollment.

Use of Services

A literature review shows that beneficiaries in the 1980s who disenrolled from HMOs had high costs; this is still true in the 1990s. Analysis of Medicare spending during 1989–1994 for beneficiaries who left HMOs shows that six months later their costs were 160 percent of fee-for-service average costs. These findings were fairly uniform across market areas and types of HMOs (Nelson et al. 1996). When adjusted for factors included in the AAPCC, the differential fell to a still substantial 42 percent. This may reflect some "pent up" need for care, but it certainly also indicates substantial adverse selection of disenrollees.

A GAO study analyzed 1992 fee-for-service expenditures for beneficiaries who enrolled in HMOs in 1993 and 1994 and compared the group that disenrolled within six months with those who remained enrolled (USGAO 1997). The disenrollees had preenrollment expenditures that were on average 79 percent higher than the continuous enrollees; $329 per month compared with $184 per month. Prior expenditures have reasonably high predictive value for future expenditures for people with chronic conditions (Kronick, Lee, and Zhou 1996).

A Florida study found that disenrollees used health services in the months after disenrolling more intensively than beneficiaries who remained in managed care (Morgan et al. 1997).[11] In addition, billing and enrollment records for Florida Medicare recipients between 1990 and 1993 showed that, in the year before enrollment, disenrollees from HMOs had only two-thirds the use of inpatient services of a matched group of Medicare beneficiaries in fee-for-service but used 180 percent more inpatient hospital services during the three months after disenrolling. The differences were consistent (although with variable magnitudes) when the sample was disaggregated by age, race, gender, and income (above/below $15,000).

To summarize so far, although rates have fallen since the early days of Medicare risk contracting, there is still considerable disenrollment, and it is selective of higher risk people. Beneficiaries who switch from one HMO to another are similar to continuous enrollees in health, functional status, attitudes, and typical health service use and demographic characteristics (Nelson et al. 1996). However, compared with enrollees who stay in their HMO and with people who switch to other HMOs, disenrollees who go into fee-for-service are much less healthy, more likely to be very old, Medicaid-eligible, and disabled, and hence present higher risks (Riley, Tudor, Chiang, and Ingber 1996; Nelson et al. 1996). Disenrollment exacerbates risk selection among Medicare HMOs relative to the fee-for-service beneficiaries.

Does a scrutiny of reasons for disenrolling provide any clues about why disenrollment exacerbates risk selection? Chapter 2 noted that disenrollment could be selective of sicker, costlier beneficiaries either because of consumer choices and systematic differences in preferences between those who need more care and those who need less, or because plans may deliberately not excel in the care of very ill and very expensive people or even try to encourage more costly enrollees to leave the plan. Involuntary disenrollment is not relevant to this discussion. Voluntary disenrollment in response to the "pull" of a more attractive alternative, and even some voluntary disenrollment attributable to "push" factors, may be related to health status but is not likely to reflect plan efforts to shed sicker people. Some voluntary disenrollment is related to provider turnover, as beneficiaries try to maintain established provider relationships. Nelson et al. (1996) found that 10 percent of switchers moved because their physician left the plan, died, or retired.[12] Changing patient needs and health status may also trigger disenrollment, even if a beneficiary has been satisfied with his or her care but wishes to receive care from a provider not available in the present plan. The question then is whether plans have adequate specialists on their panels or avoid providers who tend to attract particularly risky patients.

Much voluntary disenrollment reflects market changes (e.g., the entry of new plans or changes in plan benefits or prices). Beneficiaries are price sensitive, and even a relatively small rise in a plan's premium may trigger substantial disenrollment if there are cheaper comparable plans in the market. In the survey reported by Nelson et al. (1996), 17 percent of switchers and 10 percent of disenrollees to fee-for-service said they disenrolled primarily to get better benefits or lower costs. To the extent that sicker people have stronger ties to physicians, they are less likely to move in response to market changes. However, in some markets—for example, in California where there are a number of competing HMOs and many physicians and physician groups have multiple participation—beneficiaries may be able to switch HMOs without changing their providers. This can lead to "ping pong" —switching from one HMO to another by beneficiaries who have reached their benefit limits. For example, if plans all provide drugs up to a limit of

$1,000 per year, beneficiaries may change HMOs when they reach the drug limit to be able to get drug benefits from a new HMO.

Disenrollment that is triggered by dissatisfaction, perceptions of poor service, or denial of necessary care raises flags because it may point to efforts by plans to shed sicker, riskier enrollees. Dissatisfaction accounts for a substantial part of all disenrollment. In the 1996 survey, about 40 percent of disenrollees to fee-for-service and one-third of the plan switchers cited access to care and other problems with their plans or physicians as the main reason for leaving (Nelson et al. 1996). This is in the same ballpark as other surveys; for example, 41 percent of 375 disenrollees surveyed as part of the 1984 evaluation of the Competition Demonstration left because they were dissatisfied with some aspect of the service received in their HMO, and 43 percent of disenrollees in Harrington et al.'s survey reported dissatisfaction with physicians or medical care, including access to appropriate treatment and tests, as a major reason for disenrollment (Tucker and Langwell 1988; Harrington, Newcomer, and Preston 1993).[13]

There is no statistical evidence, but there are anecdotes about plans actively encouraging high-risk beneficiaries to disenroll. A former executive director of the Center for Health Care Rights in Los Angeles testified before the Senate Special Committee on Aging in 1995 that there was a pattern of HMO denials of home healthcare services in California and that "HMOs have told enrollees or family members that they might be able to obtain home health services if they disenroll from the HMO and rejoin the fee-for-service system just to discourage appeals and encourage high-cost patients to disenroll" (Dallek 1995). This is a long way from evidence of widespread actions by plans to induce selective disenrollment. However, the considerable evidence that disenrollment is selective of sicker people implies, at the very least, that some plans are not doing as good a job as they could in caring for members with higher than average needs for care.

Large variation exists in plan disenrollment rates, even within market areas. High disenrollment relative to competitors could signal problems, especially if accompanied (as is often the case) by complaints. Even where average rates are low, there can be a wide range of disenrollment rates across plans. For example, in 1995, rates ranged from 4 percent to 42 percent among HMOs in Los Angeles and 12 percent to 37 percent in Miami, while average rates for California were around 10 percent and around 25 percent for Florida (USGAO 1997; Dallek and Swirsky 1997). Efforts to explain variations have found that lower rates are associated with less competitive markets, larger enrollment, longer participation in the Medicare program, and nonprofit status. But there is much variation among plans that is not explained by any of the "structural" factors that are amenable to measurement. There is an association among low disenrollment, beneficiary satisfaction, and measures of plan quality. Six of the ten nonprofit HMO plans with the lowest disenrollment rates were also listed among *U.S. News & World Report*'s top HMOs (Dallek and Swirsky 1997). As one would expect, really good plans are more likely to retain their members. The question is whether plans whose members leave in droves or those that have a pattern of shedding particularly sick members should be "fingered" and brought to book in some way.

IS ENOUGH BEING DONE ABOUT DISENROLLMENT?

Monitoring Disenrollment and Reacting to High Rates

At present, HCFA collects monthly disenrollment data from all HMOs.[14] The number of people voluntarily disenrolling each month are tracked, with particular attention paid to "rapid disenrollees"—those who leave within three months of enrolling. If an HMO has unusually high disenrollment for its market area and high levels of complaints, this may trigger a letter or visit from the regional HCFA office to review the actions of the HMO, particularly the marketing activities. Monitoring protocols have been developed to guide the process. Where HCFA considers the actions of the plan to be problematic, the plan will be required to submit a corrective plan of action for HCFA's review and approval. HCFA may return to check the implementation of such plans. HCFA staff say that plans are usually compliant. Sanctions are rare: in the past three years, only three plans have been asked to suspend enrollment pending resolution of a problem. Such actions invariably spark media attention that generates adverse publicity that plans want to avoid.

These actions are rather limited, and the GAO, among others, has long been calling for HCFA to do more, especially to publish disenrollment data.[15] Region IX HCFA posts monthly disenrollment rates for all California Medicare HMOs on the Internet. The HCFA central office should do this for all market areas, and plans to do so in the spring of 1999. In any event, the BBA of 1997 requires that information be mailed to everyone eligible for Medicare before each November open enrollment period, including "to the extent available . . . disenrollment rates for Medicare enrollees electing to receive benefits through the plan for the previous two years (excluding disenrollment due to death or moving outside the plan's service area)" (BBA 1997, Section 4000). HCFA has been considering which disenrollment rates to calculate and make public and how to present them and expects to make decisions about this during 1998. The Medicare handbook is being revised in 1998 to include comparative plan information, and in late 1999, full beneficiary information packages will be mailed, preceding the first coordinated open enrollment period.

It is expected that beneficiaries may avoid plans with disenrollment rates well above average, and plans will have an incentive to address the causes of high disenrollment rates. Posting rates on the Internet would make them available to persons other than Medicare beneficiaries and make them available year-round.

Along with disenrollment rates, the number and type of complaints made against plans should also be published. This would provide an even stronger incentive to plans with consistently higher disenrollment and complaint rates than their competitors to understand and address the causes, lest high Medicare disenrollment and dissatisfaction make it harder for them to generate new enrollment of Medicare beneficiaries and of others. At present, no good mechanism exists for recording and collecting complaints. The ability and interest to do so varies across HCFA regional offices. It would be important to develop a uniform system for recording complaints before beginning to publish data on complaints.

The impending change in disenrollment rules mandated by the BBA complicates the decision as to which disenrollment data to publish. At present, beneficiaries may disenroll at any time from a Medicare HMO. Disenrollment is effective the first day of the month following the receipt of the request by the HMO or Social Security office. After the HMO enrollment period, which begins in November 2001, beneficiaries will be allowed to switch plans or disenroll into fee-for-service at any time during the first six months of 2002, but will then be locked in until the next November open enrollment period. From January 2003, the "open" period before the lock-in becomes effective will be shortened to three months.

There are some exceptions to the lock-in: beneficiaries will be able to disenroll "for cause" at any time, with "cause" including: a plan terminating or defaulting on its risk contract; the beneficiary moving out of the plan's area of operation; plan substantial violations of material provisions of the contract (such as denial of a covered service or failure to meet applicable quality standards); if beneficiaries have been misled during marketing or enrollment; or if individuals meet "other exceptional conditions" to be decided by the HCFA secretary. Clearly this provision is open to wide interpretation. Different rules also apply for newly eligible Medicare beneficiaries and for those who have never before been enrolled in an HMO. Beneficiaries with no history of HMO enrollment who wish to try managed care will have a guarantee of issue of four of the standard Medigap plans for the first six months after enrolling in an HMO. New eligibles will be allowed to disenroll to fee-for-service at any time during their first year of eligibility and will continue (as is now the case) to have guaranteed issue for all Medigap plans for six months after becoming eligible for Medicare.

These new provisions will obviously affect disenrollment patterns and rates. Disenrollment will become concentrated in the open enrollment period, with some "rapid disenrollment" occurring during the three months after the November open period and during the rest of year for new Medicare eligibles and others who are allowed to disenroll "for cause." This offers an opportunity for analysts to focus on beneficiary decisions taken during November and the following three months. An annual review at this time will cover most disenrollment, rather than having to monitor rates throughout the year.

It is important that when rates are published, clear explanation is provided of what the rates measure and how to interpret them.[16] Cohort disenrollment rates—the percentage of a particular cohort or group of enrollees who disenroll within three months and within 12 months—are probably the easiest to understand. They are preferable when enrollment is changing rapidly (as is currently the case) to annual disenrollment ratios, in which the number of disenrollees during the year is calculated as a percentage of total enrollment during that period. Annual ratios are affected by the size and rate of changes in enrollment because this is the denominator that is used in calculating the ratio, which affects comparisons of HMOs of different sizes or those whose enrollment is growing at very different rates. The restrictions on disenrollment in the BBA will make monthly and quarterly rates much more difficult to interpret and to compare across HMOs. In order to make disenrollment rates more useful to beneficiaries trying to choose among HMOs, it would be useful to include additional information such as the date when the HMO began participating in Medicare, total number of enrollees (Medicare and others), and the areas served by the plan.

Soliciting More Information from Disenrollees

Disenrollment rates can be a good indicator of high dissatisfaction among plan enrollees, but because there are many reasons people disenroll, it would be useful to solicit reasons from disenrollees routinely and to publish some summary of the results that indicates to beneficiaries how many enrollees leave because they are disssatisfied with the plan's performance, as opposed to other "benign" reasons. Reasons are solicited in an ad hoc way at present. The Social Security Disenrollment Form includes routine questions about beneficiary reasons for disenrolling, but the Social Security Administration does not capture this information, therefore it is not provided to HCFA. Nor is HCFA told anything about reasons for disenrolling for people who disenroll by signing the disenrollment form provided by the HMO, by notifying the HMO in writing, or by simply signing up with another plan with a Medicare contract (although many plans survey or interview their own disenrollees, this information is not made public).

There have been a number of surveys of disenrollees commissioned since the risk program began. In 1985, as part of a comprehensive evaluation of the Medicare Competition Demonstration Plans, Mathematica conducted a beneficiary survey that asked 140 people why they had disenrolled from Medicare HMOs (Brown et al. 1986). HCFA has itself commissioned one survey of disenrollees (Porell et al. 1992).[17] We have cited extensively the survey conducted by Mathematica under commission from the PPRC that questioned 559 disenrollees to fee-for-service and 431 switchers (Nelson et al. 1996).

HCFA has some plans for future surveys of disenrollees.[18] HCFA is working with the contractor on the Consumer Assessment of Health Plans Study (CAHPS) to develop a Medicare version of the disenrollee survey module, and HCFA will field the survey sometime in 1999. It will be made available to plans to use if they choose. Plans who contract with physicians who assume certain levels of financial risk are presently required to survey their enrollees and disenrollees (as part of efforts to monitor the effect on care and satisfaction of different physician incentive systems). However, there is no standard survey instrument, specific sampling and survey guidelines, or uniform reporting requirements. Plans are required only to summarize their survey findings to HCFA, without any indication of the nature or level of detail of the information to provide. Especially once the CAHPS survey instruments for Medicare are ready and tested, it would seem reasonable and efficient for HCFA to require plans to use at least some of the modules in the CAHPS survey and to report the parts of the survey results that would be particularly useful to monitor disenrollment.

An alternative strategy for getting useful information about disenrollment reasons would avoid reliance on plans as a source of information that may be highly critical of the care they provided. When the new enrollment and disenrollment rules and procedures are implemented, HCFA could require beneficiaries who wish to leave a plan to complete a short disenrollment form, which could include a few questions to elicit their reasons. This would be less expensive and quicker than the large surveys that have occasionally been done. Questions could be in the form of a short checklist, which would focus on issues that may indicate problems with the plan.

Enough is known from past surveys about the range of reasons for disenrollment to devise a simple checklist that disenrollees could be asked to use to signal disenrollment because of problems with the care the plan is providing, because of misleading marketing, or at the inducement of the plan or physicians. For example, a checklist could offer the following options to disenrollees:

❑ No real problems with existing plan, but prefer another plan or fee-for-service

❑ Physician or HMO employee advised a change (please explain who and why)

❑ Dissatisfied with plan for the following reason/s:

> ❑ Plan marketing was misleading, confusing, or provided inadequate information
>
> ❑ Care that Medicare should cover was denied or unreasonable obstacles were encountered to getting needed care (please give details)
>
> ❑ Quality of care provided was poor (please explain)

HCFA has already taken some steps in this direction. After the agreement with the SSA to process disenrollment expires at the end of 1998, HCFA may consider switching to a system where people who wish to disenroll and return to fee-for-service call a toll-free number to request a form, which would include questions of the sort suggested above. In addition, HCFA is developing a form that beneficiaries who wish to switch from one HMO to another could use, which would also capture reasons for the switch. The change to the new system of coordinated enrollment offers new opportunities, as do the demonstration projects to investigate the use of a broker to handle the enrollment process.

Making HMOs with High Disenrollment Accountable

Even aside from concerns about adverse publicity, in general plans do not want their enrollees to be dissatisfied or to disenroll. Publishing disenrollment rates and reasons may strengthen HMOs' incentives to reduce disenrollment and dissatisfaction. The risk selection concern is focused on a relatively small number of high utilizers of care. Even if HCFA were to be able to measure usefully disenrollment of this target group and were to publicize it, the effects on beneficiary enrollment decisions and hence on risk selection at enrollment may be mixed. Discovering that disenrollees from a plan are disproportionately those who are chronically ill or in greater need of care is likely to discourage enrollment of all beneficiaries, but most especially the chronically ill. Given strong financial incentives for avoiding having the sickest beneficiaries as plan members, publicizing information on selection disenrollment may be insufficient to get plans to set up care systems that encourage these people to enroll and stay enrolled, and may even have the reverse effect.

So if identifying plans whose enrollees—especially sick ones—express high levels of dissatisfaction through much higher disenrollment rates than competing plans, or complaints and publishing this information is not enough to encourage plans to serve the neediest beneficiaries well, then there are additional policy options.

Plans could be required to take corrective action. HCFA has not always acted decisively in the past when problems have been identified. For example, in Texas, PCA Health Plans had very high disenrollment and rapid disenrollment rates and was the object of numerous consumer complaints. However, it was not HCFA but the state attorney general who negotiated an agreement with PCA requiring the HMO to modify its enrollment practices.[19] It has been pointed out that HCFA's scope of activities in the managed care market has expanded dramatically recently and that the agency needs more resources to adequately implement its many initiatives and to monitor the growing number of managed care plans (Dallek 1997; USGAO 1997). HCFA's need for additional resources will become more acute, because the recent unprecedented growth in the number of plans participating in the Medicare risk program is likely to continue and even accelerate as a result of all the new plan types that the BBA authorizes to participate under the Medicare+Choice program.

Some disenrollment could be averted if there were a more streamlined process of appeal against denials of care by HMOs. A toll-free complaints number would be very helpful, with trained counselors who are able to address the matter with the plan immediately and try to resolve it before having to resort to the formal appeal process, which usually takes many months and can take up to a year. In April 1997, HCFA introduced an expedited appeals process in which beneficiary appeals of HMO denials of care or payment ("adverse organization determinations") must receive a response within 72 hours (HCFA 1997). This covers decisions that could jeopardize life, health, or ability to regain maximum function and terminations of care such as skilled nursing facility discharge. In addition, new regulations are being drafted to reduce the time within which non-expedited appeals must be processed. The plan is to reduce the present 60-day period for each step of the appeal process to 14 days. However, it is easier to mandate a standard of appeal than to ensure that it is met. The explosion in managed care enrollment is likely to increase the volume of appeals, and it may need additional staff as well as new streamlined processes to deal with complaints and appeals efficiently and quickly.

Finally, financial penalties could be levied. HCFA should systematically collect data on the post-disenrollment expenditures of beneficiaries who voluntarily disenroll from a plan to fee-for-service and compare these expenditures to the amount of capitation payment the HMO would have received if the beneficiary had stayed enrolled. If post-disenrollment expenditures are consistently higher than the capitation, a strong argument can be made that the HMO should pay for what would have been its financial responsibility if the beneficiary had remained enrolled. It would make sense to interview a sample of high-cost disenrollees to better understand their experiences and to assess the extent to which it seems fair to hold plans accountable for high post-enrollment expenditures.

Even if payments were to be adjusted to reflect enrollee health status, there would still be outliers—many beneficiaries whose healthcare costs could reasonably be expected to exceed the payments that would be made to plans that enroll them. The financial incentives to plans to avoid or shed such beneficiaries would persist, even with health-based payments. Thus, there will be a continued need to monitor the frequency and patterns of disenrollment and post-disenrollment costs so that the possibility of being identified and sanctioned will limit the incentive to plans to try to rid themselves of high-cost enrollees.

NOTES

1. Beth Kosiak provided much of the information in this chapter about HCFA's role and plans, and detailed and helpful comments, especially on the final section. The author is responsible for any remaining errors. Rick Kronick also provided very helpful comments on this chapter.
2. Recent research findings of these magnitudes are cited later in the chapter.
3. Reported disenrollment rates usually exclude beneficiaries who die while enrolled in HMOs, who lose their Part B entitlement, or who were in plans that terminated their risk contracts. This "involuntary disenrollment" affects about 3 percent of beneficiaries annually.
4. This is the only study of recent disenrollment experience that calculated rates in exactly the same way as the earlier Brown and Langwell studies to determine whether rates have changed. Brown and Langwell followed a cohort of enrollees for 12 months and measured the percentage who disenrolled within 12 months of enrolling.
5. Riley et al.'s annualized rates were calculated as 1 – [(1–January disenrollment rate)(1–February disenrollment rate)....(1–December disenrollment rate)]. That is, they multiplied monthly retention rates (1–disenrollment rates) for all 12 months and subtracted the product from 1.
6. Dallek and Swirsky calculated annual disenrollment rates by adding the number of voluntary disenrollments in each month of the year and taking this total as a percentage of average yearly membership, calculated as the sum of the end-of-the-month membership totals for the year, divided by 12.
7. The methodology used by Nelson et al. underestimates disenrollment compared to the other studies cited. Confining the sample of enrollees to those who had been enrolled for at least two months excludes many so-called "rapid disenrollees" who disenroll within three months. Furthermore, although Nelson et al.'s measure of the incidence of disenrollment during a 12-month snapshot includes people who had enrolled prior to the study

period and disenrolled during the sampled year, it misses those who disenrolled after the study period.

8. This is the most recent, and largest survey of disenrollees, and was commissioned by the PPRC. Harrington et al. (1993) review a number of earlier surveys, citing Rossiter et al. (1988, 1989); Tucker and Langwell (1989); Ward (1987); Langwell and Hadley (1989); Mechanic et al. (1983); and Sorenson and Wersinger (1981).

9. The five chronic conditions were diabetes mellitus, ischemic heart disease, congestive heart failure, hypertension, and chronic obstructive pulmonary disease. California accounted for one-third of all Medicare HMO enrollment in 1995.

10. Adjustments were made for age and sex.

11. The sample size was 375,406 beneficiaries in fee-for-service, 48,380 enrollees before enrollment and 23,879 disenrollees. The study also found that higher use of services after disenrollment declined after six months, and reenrollment in a managed care plan tended to occur at about the time that hospital admission rates approximated that of fee-for-service Medicare beneficiaries.

12. This was the main reason for leaving for only 1.2 percent of disenrollees who changed to fee-for-service.

13. We have excluded from the "dissatisfied" category used by Tucker and Langwell those who said they disenrolled because the HMO was too expensive or because they heard of a better plan, because of the distinction we have drawn between negative "push" factors and the "pull" of a more attractive alternative. Harrington, Newcomer, and Preston (1993) interviewed 473 people who had been enrolled for at least 12 months, but who disenrolled between June 1987 and September 1988 from four plans participating in a HCFA demonstration program known as Social/HMOs, in which plans provided expanded and chronic care benefits in addition to the standard Medicare package. They report "main reasons" for disenrollment (allowing respondents to cite more than one), whereas the other studies cited here elicited a single main reason.

14. Information on HCFA's current efforts from Rae Lowen, HCFA, personal communication.

15. For example, USGAO (1996) called for disenrollment and complaints and appeals data to be published. Other GAO reports reiterate this suggestion.

16. HCFA recognizes that some changes are needed in the way some rates are computed, notably that rapid disenrollment ought to be computed as a percentage of new enrollees, not of total enrollment, as in the past. Rae Lowen, HCFA, personal communication 5/97.

17. This survey used data from 1989–90 (personal communication, Beth Kosiak, HCFA 3/3/98). HCFA seems to have intended to do periodic surveys and had developed a disenrollee survey instrument which Langwell et al. (1989) include as Appendix A.

18. Telephone communication with Beth Kosiak, HCFA, June 1997.

19. In re Texas v. PCA Health Plans of Texas, Inc., Texas District Court, 353 Judicial District, No. 9712378, 11/3/97.

REFERENCES

Brown, R., K. Langwell, K. Berman, A. Ciemnecki, L. Nelson, A. Schreier, and A. Tucker. 1986. *Enrollment and Disenrollment in Medicare Competition Demonstration Plans: A Descriptive Analysis.* Princeton, NJ: Mathematica Policy Research Inc.

Dallek, G. 1995. www.tahc.org. February 18, 1998.

Dallek, G. 1997. *Medicare Managed Care: Securing Beneficiary Protections.* Washington, DC: Families USA Foundation.

Dallek, G., and L. Swirsky. 1997. *Comparing Medicare HMOs: Do They Keep Their Members?* Washington, DC: Families USA Foundation.

Harrington, C., R. Newcomer, and S. Preston. 1993. "A Comparison of S/HMO Disenrollees and Continuing Members." *Inquiry* 30 (4): 429–40.

Health Care Financing Administration (HCFA). 1997. "Managed Care in Medicare and Medicaid." Fact Sheet. http://www.hcfa.gov/facts/f960900.htm.

Kronick, R., L. Lee, and Z. Zhou. 1996. "Diagnostic Risk Adjustment for Medicaid: The Disability Payment System." *Health Care Financing Review* 17 (3): 7–34.

Langwell, K. M., and J. P. Hadley. 1989. "Evaluation of the Medicare Competition Demonstrations." *Health Care Financing Review* 11 (2): 65–80.

Langwell, K. M., S. Stearns, S. Nelson, J. Bergeron, L. Schopler, and R. Donahey. 1989. *Disenrollment Experience in the TEFRA HMO/CMP Program, 1985 to 1988.* Washington, DC: Mathematica Policy Research Inc.

Mechanic, D., N. Weiss, and P. Cleary. 1983. "The Growth of HMOs: Issues of Enrollment and Disenrollment." *Medical Care* 21 (3): 338–47.

Morgan, R. O., B. A. Virnig, C. A. DeVito, and N. A. Persily. 1997. "The Medicare-HMO Revolving Door—The Healthy Go In and the Sick Go Out." *New England Journal of Medicine* 337 (3): 169–75.

Nelson, L., M. Gold, R. Brown, A. B. Ciemnecki, A. Aizer, and K. A. CyBulski. 1996. *Access to Care in Medicare Managed Care: Results from a 1996 Survey of Enrollees and Disenrollees.* Washington, DC: Physician Payment Review Commission.

Porell, F., C. Cocotas, P. Perales, C. Tompkins, and M. Glavin. 1992. "Factors Associated with Disenrollment from Medicare HMOs: Findings from a Survey of Disenrollees." Report prepared for HCFA. Boston: Institute for Health Policy, Brandeis University.

Riley, G., C. Tudor, Y. Chiang, and M. Ingber. 1996. "Health Status of Medicare Enrollees in HMOs and Fee-for-Service in 1994." *Health Care Financing Review* 17 (4): 65–73.

Riley, G., E. Feuer, and J. Lubitz. 1996. "Disenrollment of Medicare Cancer Patients from Health Maintenance Organizations." *Medical Care* 34 (8): 826–36.

Riley, G., M. Ingber, and C. Tudor. 1997. "Disenrollment of Medicare Beneficiaries from HMOs." *Health Affairs* 16 (5): 117–24.

Riley, G., E. Rabey, and J. Kasper. 1989. "Biased Selection and Regression toward the Mean in Three Medicare HMO Demonstrations: A Survival Analysis of Enrollees and Disenrollees." *Medical Care* 27 (4): 337–51.

Riley, G., J. Lubitz, and E. Rabey. 1991. "Enrollee Health Status under Medicare Risk Contracts: An Analysis of Mortality Rates." *Health Services Research* 26 (2): 137–63.

Rossiter, L., K. Langwell, T. Wan, and M. Rivnyak. 1989. "Patient Satisfaction Among Elderly Enrollees and Disenrollees in Medicare HMOs, Results from the National Medicare Competition Evaluation." *Journal of the American Medical Association* 262 (1): 57–63.

Sorenson, A., and R. Wersinger. 1981. "Factors Influencing Disenrollment from an HMO." *Medical Care* 19 (7): 766–73.

Tucker, A., and K. Langwell. 1989. "Disenrollment Patterns in Medicare HMOs: A Preliminary Analysis." Washington, DC: Mathematica Policy Research.

United States General Accounting Office (USGAO). 1996. *Medicare: HCFA Should Release Data to Aid Consumers, Prompt Better HMO Performance.* GAO/HEHS-97-23. Washington, DC.

United States General Accounting Office (USGAO). 1997. *Medicare: Fewer and Lower Cost Beneficiaries with Chronic Conditions Enroll in HMOs.* Report to the Chairman, Subcommittee of Health, Committee on Ways and Means, House of Representatives. GAO/HEHS-97-160. Washington, DC.

Ward, R. 1987. "HMO Satisfaction and Understanding Among Recent Medicare Enrollees." *Journal of Health and Social Behavior* 28 (4): 401–12.

Strategies to Limit Risk Selection in the Medicare Program, and Implementation Feasibility

Richard Kronick and Joy de Beyer

T
he Balanced Budget Act (BBA) of 1997 has defined an ambitious
program of reform for Medicare, introducing the most sweeping
changes in the history of the Medicare program. In addition, other
initiatives such as the Consumer Bill of Rights and recent changes in HCFA's
dispute resolution process address some of the problems with Medicare
HMOs that analysts, policymakers, and beneficiaries have raised. This chapter highlights some of the key provisions of the reform initiatives already
under way. Then it summarizes the suggestions made in the preceding chapters in this volume and discusses the feasibility of implementing them.

MEDICARE'S FUTURE: THE CURRENT REFORM AGENDA

The BBA introduces a long list of far-reaching changes in the Medicare
program. Those changes with the greatest potential for changing the program and that make the greatest administrative demands on HCFA are
changes in the payment system for managed care plans; annual provision of
comparative information to beneficiaries; coordinated open enrollment in
the Medicare+Choice program; and opening Medicare contracting to new

types of plans (in addition to HMOs) without any requirement to limit Medicare beneficiaries as a percentage of total enrollment.

The BBA mandates that health-based payment begin in 2000, but it specifies little about implementation. HCFA's current plans are to use diagnostic information from inpatient hospital stays to measure health status. This approach is a good beginning; compared to the status quo, it should make HMOs more willing to serve beneficiaries with greater than average needs. However, implementation of even this modest first step in health-based payment is threatened by political obstacles and the need for administrative resources to process inpatient diagnostic information.

Beginning in 1999, HCFA is required to annually provide beneficiaries with comparative information on all available Medicare+Choice plans in their area. This information will include side-by-side benefit and cost comparisons, as well as, to the extent available, quality measures and disenrollment rates. This information will make it much easier for beneficiaries to understand the range of choices open to them and could encourage people who previously did not realize that there were options besides traditional fee-for-service Medicare and Medigap supplements to take advantage of the richer benefit packages and lower charges that are typical of managed care plans (discussed in detail in Chapter 4).

Better information may reduce favorable selection to HMOs for two reasons. People without supplementary insurance who learn of the existence of HMOs in their area may be encouraged to try managed care, especially if zero or low premium plans are available. Among those without supplementary insurance, the financial benefits of joining an HMO will be greater for the sick than for the healthy. Second, Medigap policyholders who see price/benefit comparisons with substantially cheaper managed care plans, which perhaps even offer a richer benefit package, might well switch to HMOs. Even if their established provider relationships continue to make sicker people more reluctant to change, the switchers may well be a less favorably selected group than present HMO enrollees.

To the extent that HCFA provides information on consumer satisfaction, health plan quality, and disenrollment rates, this information may also help reduce risk selection problems for two reasons. If HMOs in a market perform well on these measures, particularly for those who are most in need of care, knowledge of this performance is likely to encourage those with higher need to switch into plans, reducing the extent of favorable selection. Publicizing information on satisfaction and quality, particularly focused on the sick, should encourage HMOs to improve their performance, which will then further reduce selection bias. The extent to which HMOs will want to look good depends in part on successful implementation of health-based payment and, in part, on questions about HMO and beneficiary choice behavior for which we do not have definitive answers. Although plans may not want to gain a reputation as being the best plan in town for beneficiaries who are really sick, they will also want to avoid getting a reputation as the worst. Even relatively healthy Medicare beneficiaries are more likely than younger persons to understand their own vulnerabilities and are likely to be reluctant to enroll in a plan with a middling to poor rating on quality and access for those most in need. Given a desire to avoid being seen as a poorly performing plan, we would expect that better information to beneficiaries on the performance of plans in caring for the vulnerable would encourage plans to improve their performance.

Also in 1999, annual coordinated open enrollment for all options in the Medicare+Choice program will begin. After a transitional phase-in year, there will be a three-month window from January through March during which beneficiaries will be able to reconsider their enrollment decision and after which (with the exceptions noted in Chapter 5 and Chapter 8) they will be locked into the plan they have chosen until the next annual enrollment period. Medigap plans are not to be included in the open enrollment system, nor did the BBA include any significant changes in the rules and procedures under which Medigap policies are sold. No attempt was made to distance plans from marketing and enrollment, except for requiring a demonstration project to experiment with using a broker for these functions.

The fourth major set of changes opens Medicare contracting to new types of non-HMO plans and relaxes the so-called "50-50 rule" so that Medicare beneficiaries are no longer limited to half of a plan's total enrollee base. This will enable the entry of smaller and new types of provider service networks into the Medicare managed care market, with potentially large implications for HCFA's regulatory and oversight burden.

Collectively, these changes are likely to introduce considerable instability—perhaps even confusion—into the Medicare program. Further, the administrative, technical, and political resources of HCFA will be sorely tested as it attempts to implement the plethora of changes mandated by the BBA, and many observers would not be surprised if some of the mandates were implemented poorly or not at all. However, the BBA is a response to changes that were already well under way: the substantial increase in managed care enrollment in Medicare (and the Congressional desire to expand this enrollment further) creates the need to make significant changes in the regulation and administration of the Medicare program in order to better protect the interests of beneficiaries.

In addition to the BBA, other healthcare reform initiatives and legislation have also mandated changes in the rules and administration of the Medicare program. The intent is to promote and assure patient protections and healthcare quality, especially in light of the growing role of managed care in Medicare. The most important initiative is the Consumer Bill of Rights and Responsibilities, which was proposed in March 1997 by the Presidential Advisory Commission on Consumer Protection and Quality in the Health Care Industry. The Commission was appointed by President Clinton in September 1996 to review the rapid changes in healthcare financing and delivery systems and to make recommendations on how to improve the nation's healthcare system. It includes Medicare within a much broader mandate. An Executive Order requires all federal healthcare programs to comply with the Consumer Bill of Rights. Many of the Bill of Rights stipulations are already met under HCFA regulations for Medicare HMOs or are covered under the BBA reforms of Medicare.

For example, the Consumer Bill of Rights states that consumers have the right to receive accurate, easily understood information and notes that some consumers require assistance in making informed healthcare decisions about their health plans, professionals, and facilities. The list of the information that ought to be provided is consistent with the BBA requirements for beneficiary information about Medicare+Choice options.

The Bill of Rights also states that "consumers have the right to a fair and efficient process for resolving differences with their health plans, health care providers, and the institutions that serve them." Until recently, Medicare dispute resolution methods have proved slow and suboptimally responsive (Dallek 1997). Plans have dragged their heels or failed to follow required procedures with impunity. Recognition of this problem and of the extreme vulnerability of beneficiaries—especially gravely ill people—has spurred the introduction of an expedited review process for Medicare beneficiaries enrolled in HMOs. The new rules were published on April 30, 1997, and Medicare contracting health plans were required to be in compliance with all requirements beginning August 28, 1997. Under the new rules, beneficiaries may appeal decisions that could jeopardize life, health, or ability to regain maximum function, and terminations of care such as skilled nursing facility discharge (but not other decisions or denial of payment) and request expedited review. For eligible decisions, plans must respond within 72 hours, and all appeals that are denied must be reported to HCFA's contractor, the Center for Dispute Resolution, which has ten days to review the HMO's decision (with an extension allowed to gather more information or conduct tests if it is in the interests of the beneficiary). New regulations are also being developed to cut the time allowed for each stage of the normal appeal process from 60 to 14 days. These changes are expected to fix one of the major failings of the Medicare HMO appeals process.

Many beneficiaries have been reluctant to join HMOs because they fear that their access to specialists will be restricted to an unacceptable degree. The Consumer Bill of Rights says that "consumers with complex or serious medical conditions who require frequent specialty care should have direct access to a qualified specialist of their choice within a plan's network of providers. Authorizations, when required, should be for an adequate number of direct access visits under an approved treatment plan." Further, plans must comply with a "provider network adequacy" clause "to ensure that all covered services will be accessible without unreasonable delay, including access to emergency services 24 hours a day and 7 days a week. If a health plan has an insufficient number or type of providers to provide a covered benefit with the appropriate degree of specialization, the plan should ensure that the consumer obtains the benefit outside the network at no greater cost than if the benefit were obtained from participating providers." If Medicare beneficiaries find these assurances credible, a substantial deterrent to joining a managed care plan may have been removed.

Finally, the Physician Incentive Rule, which became effective at the beginning of 1997, was designed to make sure that the incentives inherent in managed care to discourage unnecessary services do not go too far. Plans are required to disclose physician financial incentives at the request of beneficiaries and to ensure that no more than 25 percent of a physician's income is at risk under capitation. The regulations also ban any incentive arrangements that induce doctors to limit or reduce medically necessary services.

Together these initiatives constitute a formidable agenda for change for Medicare. To the extent that these changes, singly or severally, make HMOs more attractive—especially to beneficiaries who need higher than average levels of care—they ought to reduce the extent of favorable risk selection that HMOs have enjoyed relative to fee-for-service Medicare. The extent that this proves to be the case remains to be seen. Beneficiary response to the changes is not predictable, and plans will still have a strong incentive to try to attract healthier beneficiaries and avoid (and perhaps even evade) the sickest and most costly.[1] Moreover, in some cases, we believe that the BBA has defined partial reforms where bolder and more far-reaching changes would have been better. This volume has therefore carefully examined aspects of the Medicare program and the proposed changes in the BBA and made some additional suggestions intended to help deal with risk selection, its associated additional financial burden on the public purse, and concerns about the quality of care available to those who most need healthcare.

ADDING TO THE AGENDA: OUR SUGGESTIONS SUMMARIZED

Formidable and fine though it is, the reform agenda for Medicare established by the BBA and other new regulations still leaves gaps that could undermine the ability of the Medicare program to fulfill its mission of providing access to good quality healthcare to all eligible beneficiaries. Moreover, many details are left unspecified that need to be considered and decided. For example, the BBA requires beneficiaries to be given certain categories of information, but a huge amount of work needs to be done to decide exactly what information to provide and how best to present it. This section summarizes the key suggestions made in the preceding six chapters that either add to or elaborate on the existing reform agenda.

Better Health-Based Payment Adjustors for HMOs

HCFA plans to begin health-based payment using data from inpatient hospital stays, and we strongly support this effort as a valuable starting point. Assuming that HCFA successfully takes this first step, we recommend two additional steps that should further increase the willingness of health plans to serve the chronically ill and lead to improvements in the care that these beneficiaries receive. First, it is important to move quickly to expand the assessment of health status to the use of diagnoses made in both inpatient and ambulatory settings, as has been done recently by a number of state Medicaid programs. Relying solely on inpatient diagnoses penalizes those plans that have worked aggressively to move care out of the hospital into the community and creates incentives for plans to reengineer healthcare delivery to focus more on inpatient care. Relying only on inpatient data provides little assurance in the long run that plans with sicker members will be paid appropriately. Adding diagnostic information from ambulatory care to the assessment of health status will increase the reporting burden on plans, will increase the administrative burden on HCFA, and will increase the need to measure and adjust for accuracy in diagnostic reporting. However, the benefits from fostering the development of high quality, efficient systems of care and rewarding the plans that attract those most in need should far outweigh the costs.

Second, paying plans for high quality end-of-life care offers a simple method of health-based payment that HCFA should adopt as a supplement to the use of diagnostic information in health status assessment. Policymakers may be concerned that adjusting payments to plans based on the number of beneficiaries who die may appear to be "paying for death" and may create the wrong incentives and negative publicity. However, if HCFA develops a system for measuring the quality of care for those who die (including demonstration of improved communication between caregivers and patients/ families) and pays plans only for high quality end-of-life care, such a system could be expected to lead to substantial improvements in care for the terminally ill.

Better Information to Beneficiaries, Including Information on Medigap Options

The BBA requirement that beneficiaries be provided annually with comprehensive comparative information on their managed care choices is an excellent step toward addressing two problems: the severe information gap that beneficiaries face in knowing what options are available to them and weighing their choices, and the opportunities that individual companies and their agents have had as the main information source, for subtle (or blatant) filtering or shading of information, despite HCFA monitoring of marketing materials. However, the BBA still leaves a hole in the information by not requiring that Medigap options be included in the beneficiary information package. We believe they should be.

It is important that the information on beneficiary choices be presented in the context of a basic explanation of how Medicare works, the gaps in coverage of the basic fee-for-service program, how managed care differs from fee-for-service, and the function of supplementary insurance, because many beneficiaries have a poor understanding of the program and are unaware of the choices open to them. Difficult decisions need to be made about what information to include and how to present it. Focus group and survey research has revealed that beneficiaries give priority to comparative information on costs, coverage and exclusions, and how different systems and plans operate. They want clear explanations of rules and procedures, especially with respect to choosing providers and procedures for gaining access to specialists, emergency, after-hours, and out-of-area care. Some information on plan performance would be valued, especially regarding access to care and services and the interpersonal and technical skills of providers. Most beneficiaries are interested primarily in information that is specifically relevant to themselves. In order to get this information, it must be easy for beneficiaries to seek additional, more specific information than would make sense to provide to everyone. The volume and type of information presented and the way it is organized will affect the degree to which it facilitates beneficiaries' decision making, rather than complicates it. Great care must be taken in selecting and presenting information and in devising ways to help beneficiaries use the information. Adequate resources should be devoted to doing this well, to ensure that the information provided is what beneficiaries need to make well-informed choices.

Coordinated Annual Open Enrollment

While welcoming the new coordinated open enrollment system to be introduced for Medicare+Choice plans, Rice recommends two improvements on the BBA: that Medigap policies be included in the new annual coordinated open guaranteed enrollment system; and that a common premium rating system be adopted for HMOs and Medigap insurers (Chapter 5).

Including Medigap policies with managed care plans in an annual guaranteed open enrollment period would be a great improvement on the BBA reform, which applies only to Medicare+Choice plans. If the two parts of the Medicare market were brought into the same system, under the same set of procedures and rules regarding guaranteed issue, preexisting condition exclusions, and premium rating practices, competition would be sharpened and it would become less risky for beneficiaries to try managed care. A unified system that included Medigap policies as well managed care would provide beneficiaries with complete information about the full range of their choices within Medicare and would encourage them to think about all of their options once a year. Satisfied beneficiaries would not need to do anything; others could weigh options and make informed choices without fearing that they were burning any bridges that they might later wish to cross back over. An added advantage would be that beneficiaries would be less likely to purchase duplicative coverage under this system.

The BBA provides some reassurance to beneficiaries who wish to try managed care for the first time by allowing them guaranteed issue of some Medigap plans for six months. The proposal in this volume would provide guaranteed issue of at least some (if not all) of the available Medigap plans annually to all beneficiaries, which would be even more effective in reducing risk selection to HMOs by encouraging people—including sicker people who are likely to be warier of a change—to try an HMO without fear of not being able to regain Medigap coverage if they did not like the HMO.

Marketing Reforms

Medicare plans are presently prohibited from door-to-door and other direct marketing to individuals unless invited, and HCFA reviews plan marketing materials before they are distributed. HCFA ought to require that plan marketing materials provide specific standardized information about benefits, costs, exclusions, and rules in a consistent standardized format and use specified terminology. This would greatly simplify comparisons and facilitate compilation of comparative material.

The present focus of marketing oversight is to ensure that beneficiaries are not enticed or induced unreasonably to join (for example, enrollment gifts are prohibited). Merlis suggests two additional activities to monitor whether plans are trying to discourage enrollment of high-risk beneficiaries, which could have a significant impact on risk selection. First, he proposes adding to current oversight efforts of marketing materials by using focus groups to understand what messages beneficiaries are absorbing and the effect of marketing on different types of beneficiaries—for example, comparing high-risk and low-risk people. Second, periodic surveys of people who make contact with plan representatives but decide not to enroll would provide HCFA the opportunity to understand their decisions and discover whether sicker people were being actively or subtly discouraged.

Although plans will no longer be the only source of information for most beneficiaries once HCFA begins providing comparative information, the BBA stops far short of prohibiting plans from all face-to-face or other direct marketing. There is little evidence concerning the extent to which HMO marketing activities cause favorable selection, and hence less firm grounds for arguing that plans should be prohibited from marketing altogether, as some states have done for Medicaid. Merlis and Rice both favor the use of independent brokers or agents to handle all contact with beneficiaries pertaining to marketing and enrollment, with plans being removed entirely from these functions; the BBA requires demonstration projects to explore the role of a broker (Chapter 4). Mindful of the extent to which plans would likely resist being removed from marketing and enrollment, Rice suggests a second best but pragmatic option of adding independent brokers as a second method of enrollment. Beneficiaries would be able to choose between enrolling directly with plans or through independent brokers who would provide the necessary information, answer questions, and process HMO enrollment. Enrollment through a third-party broker would have two advantages: convenience for beneficiaries who may want to enroll after receiving information on their options from a broker; and the removal of one opportunity for plans to discourage high-risk beneficiaries from enrolling. The possible disadvantages are the cost, confusion from dual sources of enrollment, the risk that brokers may not do a good job of explaining HMO exclusions, rules and procedures, and possible delays in HMOs learning that beneficiaries have enrolled. We think that these potential drawbacks would be outweighed by the advantages.

Reduce Benefit Package Diversity

The BBA makes no attempt to reduce the variety in HMO benefit packages on offer. Two kinds of problems arise if beneficiaries are asked to choose among HMOs that offer highly varied benefit packages. First, it is difficult for beneficiaries to make an informed choice among plans, because price differences may reflect variations in quality and efficiency as well as variations in covered benefits. Uncertainty about judging value will likely reduce the rewards to those provider groups that in fact are good at creating value. Second, allowing diversity in benefit packages invites plans to attempt to segment the market and select risks.

Many large employers require each HMO to offer virtually the same set of covered benefits and the same copayment structure. This requirement facilitates comparison across plans and is thought to have sharpened competition among HMOs and led to restraint in price growth. Although theoretically an option for HCFA as well, a uniform HMO benefit package is not practical because Medicare beneficiaries are a large and heterogeneous group, with wide diversity in the kinds and levels of coverage that they prefer, and because premiums and packages differ substantially across the country. Consider, for example, the extent of prescription drug coverage. If HCFA mandated that all HMOs offer only one package to Medicare beneficiaries, and that package included prescription drug coverage at, for example, the level of Medigap policy J,[2] then in many areas of the country HMOs would need to charge a relatively high premium for this plan. This premium could price low-income beneficiaries out of the HMO market. These beneficiaries would be forced to stay in fee-for-service and pay copayments and deductibles when they might prefer a lower option HMO plan; further, it would discourage some from switching from Medigap policy C—which does not cover drugs—into the HMO, even when the HMO may be a better value for them if it excluded drug coverage. Conversely, if the HCFA-mandated package did not include prescription drugs, then beneficiaries living in Southern California and other areas where drugs are included today in zero premium plans would be worse off.

The best compromise between maintaining choices in benefit packages and the benefits of standardization would be to establish a limited and well-defined set of supplemental benefits packages that HMOs would be allowed to offer. The set of packages should be as close as possible to the set of Medigap supplements, to facilitate comparison between HMOs and Medigap. The set of packages could be established by HCFA, after consultation with beneficiaries, the HMOs serving Medicare beneficiaries, and the NAIC. This would leave the choice environment more confusing than the environment facing many privately insured, but substantially less chaotic than the current environment. If the supplemental benefits offered by HMOs were limited to a set of packages from a predetermined list, then beneficiaries would be able to compare prices more easily across plans and more easily compare prices and benefits between HMOs and Medigap policies.

The main disadvantage of a prescribed list for supplemental benefits compared to the status quo is that it inhibits innovation and responsiveness to changes in consumer preferences: if an HMO were to figure out a new benefit that it wanted to offer and that beneficiaries might value highly, it would be prohibited from doing so. However, there has been a prescribed list of supplemental benefits for Medigap policies since 1990, and there is little evidence or suggestion that this restriction has caused problems.

The disadvantage of a prescribed list compared to a single benefit package is the concern that risk-selection dynamics will cause the more generous packages on the list to be priced at well above their actuarial value, much higher than if enrollment were not biased. The more sensitive health-based payment that Kronick and Dreyfus advocate would ameliorate this problem to some extent. Further, at least in areas of the country where the AAPCC is well above the amount that HMOs need to provide basic Medicare coverage, only benefit packages that are more expansive than the packages that efficient plans can offer for zero premium would be likely to be affected.

Doing More to Ensure Good Quality Care, Especially for Beneficiaries Most in Need

A number of state Medicaid programs have established selection criteria for HMOs serving Medicaid recipients with disability that are designed to increase the likelihood that the plans will actually do a good job of serving those recipients most in need. These criteria include requirements in the following areas:

- HMOs must perform an initial assessment for all new enrollees to identify beneficiaries with chronic health problems.
- For all chronically ill enrollees, a plan of care must be produced (preferably by a multi-disciplinary team) that should include discussion of anticipated needs for home health and durable medical equipment and consideration of the need for mental health services.
- A system must be in place for 24-hour telephone access to medical advice.
- HMOs must conduct (and report to the Medicaid agency) the results of a specified number (e.g., five) of quality improvement initiatives each year; some of these initiatives may be in areas chosen by the agency and uniform across plans; others may be chosen by the plans.
- HMOs must conduct health education and prevention programs that target the needs of the chronically ill.
- HMOs must report on the processes employed to decide on the use of home health, durable medical equipment, and mental health services, the extent to which these services are used, and the number and disposition of beneficiary complaints about these services.
- HMOs must have a member services representative to help link beneficiaries with community-based organizations.

HCFA already has licensing and other requirements that HMOs participating in Medicare risk contracts must fulfill. We think that carefully devised additional requirements could help ensure that participating HMOs are more responsive to the needs of disabled and chronically ill beneficiaries. However, it would be no easy task to decide which requirements would be most effective or to find a single set of requirements appropriate for all Medicare HMOs.

The suggested focus on health plan process measures is needed because our ability to measure and report on health plan quality is still rudimentary. There are already several major initiatives under way to monitor and report on quality of care. For managed care, a good beginning is being made with the standardized satisfaction surveys of HMO enrollees (known as the Consumer Assessment of Health Plans Study, or CAHPS, survey) being administered to beneficiaries in all plans that have had active risk contracts for at least a year and with the requirement that HMOs produce HEDIS reports. But there is still a long way to go, including difficulty in producing good comparative information on quality of care in fee-for-service. A useful addition to ongoing efforts would be a systematic review of a sample of deaths, both among HMO enrollees and from fee-for-service, as discussed in Chapter 3.

Monitoring Disenrollment

Disenrollment is selective of sicker beneficiaries, and in the months after disenrolling, beneficiaries who disenroll into fee-for-service incur much higher healthcare expenditures than other beneficiaries in fee-for-service. It is not possible, based on existing evidence, to judge the extent to which (if it all) plans contribute to selective disenrollment by inducing the sickest or potentially most costly beneficiaries to disenroll. We therefore propose that HCFA institute routine "exit poll" surveys of disenrollees to investigate the reasons for disenrollment. Disenrollment reasons—appropriately categorized—should be published, because they are useful information for beneficiaries making enrollment decisions. HCFA should also collect data on the post-disenrollment expenditures of beneficiaries who disenroll from a plan to fee-for-service, and compare these expenditures to the amount of capitation payment the HMO would have received if the beneficiary had stayed enrolled. If, on average, post-enrollment expenditures are higher than the capitation, then corrective action should be considered, such as requiring the plan to pay for what would have been its financial responsibility if the beneficiary had remained enrolled.

FEASIBILITY

Several factors affect the feasibility of reforms: (a) cost; (b) whether legislative change would be needed, and if so whether it would have an easy passage through the legislative process; (c) whether the proposed action would be generally accepted as an appropriate role for a public bureaucracy; (d) whether adequate experience and expertise exist to guide implementation in the Medicare program; and (e) the extent to which vested interests are likely to generate opposition.

Table 9.1 summarizes our assessment of the feasibility of each of the key proposals made in this volume. We have used a simple scoring system: 0 indicates "no problem," a 1 indicates that the factor listed in the column (cost, legislation needed, etc.) would pose a problem in implementing the proposal, and a 2 indicates a factor that would be highly problematic for a particular proposal. A final column contains our opinion on the extent to which the action would be likely to reduce risk selection, using a 3-point scoring system: * for a small impact, ** for a moderate impact, and *** for a substantial impact. We also prioritize our suggestions, giving highest priority to actions that are likely to make a real difference to risk selection problems and that would not face formidable barriers to implementation.

Given the fiscal imperative to contain Medicare expenditures, cost considerations weigh heavily. We have not attempted to quantify the likely costs of implementing our proposals. However, even the most expensive is likely to be small compared to the cost of risk selection to HCFA: favorable selection is estimated to have cost Medicare at least $2.2 billion in the last three years. If the proposed changes reduced favorable selection to HMOs significantly (as we expect they would) they could potentially easily pay for themselves, as well as increase quality and access for those beneficiaries most in need.

The potential effect of some of the proposed actions on risk selection is partly dependent on being able to achieve other changes. For example, including Medigap information provided to beneficiaries would have a much larger impact on risk selection if combined with guaranteed annual enrollment in Medigap. Then beneficiaries would be apprised of the full range of their options and could try managed care knowing that they could regain their Medigap coverage if they wished the following year. Table 9.1 does not capture these sorts of synergies and "interaction effects" among the various proposals.

This chapter and Table 9.1 summarize approximately a dozen actions that the book suggests should be added to the reform agenda with which HCFA is already grappling. Even in the most optimistic of possible worlds, one has to decide what to tackle first. Given the realistic recognition that time and other resource constraints as well as legislative, technical, and political barriers severely limit what is likely to be accomplished, we have prioritized these suggestions. At the top of the list are the things that are likely to do much to address risk selection and the associated problems and that appear to have the best chance of being implemented successfully.

Table 9.1 Factors Affecting Feasibility of Proposals

Proposal	Cost to HCFA	New Legislation	Appropriate and acceptable HCFA role?	Can it be done effectively?	Would vested interests be threatened?	Likely impact on risk selection problems?
Health-based payment	1	0	0	1	2	***
Devote adequate resources to research and testing to ensure that information on benefits, premiums, plan quality, and enrollee satisfaction meets needs well	2	0	0	1 or 2	1	***
Medigap						
(a) Include Medigap in beneficiary information	1	0	0	0	1	*
(b) Include Medigap in the guaranteed coordinated annual open enrollment	0	1	1	0	2	***
(c) Adopt common premium rating system for HMOs and Medigap insurers	0	1	1	0	2	**
Require standardized marketing information from plans	0	0	0	0	0	*

Continued

Table 9.1 (continued)

Proposal	Cost to HCFA	New Legislation	Appropriate and acceptable HCFA role?	Can it be done effectively?	Would vested interests be threatened?	Likely impact on risk selection problems?
Gather more information on market impact and reasons for not enrolling in plans	1	0	1	1	0	*
Independent enrollment broker	1	2	2	1	2	Uncertain
Supplementary benefits	0	1	2	0	1	*
New service and care requirements catering to needs of disabled and chronically ill enrollees	0	0	2	2	1	***
Disenrollment						
(a) Routinely survey disenrollees to fee-for-service and publish data	1	0	0	0	0	*
(b) Monitor post-disenrollment costs for high-cost disenrollees to fee-for-service, institute financial penalties	0	1	1	1	1	*

Note: 0 signifies "no problem or minor problem"
1 signifies "significant obstacle"
2 signifies "major obstacle"

Implement Health-Based Payment

Improving the extent to which the payment system adjusts for risk as far as present technical developments and information systems allow should be the first priority. Changing the HMO payment system to pay more to plans that attract beneficiaries with greater needs is the most powerful single tool to reduce the incentive to HMOs to avoid those most in need of care. This change would do much to reduce the powerful incentive to systematically avoid high-risk people, would remove the disincentive against deserving a reputation for excellent care of very ill people, and would pay plans commensurately with the health needs of their enrollees.

The principle of adjusting payments for risk is already enshrined in the existing AAPCC system. Its inadequacies have been lamented long and loud. There is widespread approval of health-based payments, perhaps even a reasonable consensus that they are desirable. Expertise in developing and implementing these systems is growing as more and more state Medicaid programs adopt them. The information hurdle is significant but not impossible, and if plans were required to capture and report encounter data, they might start to analyze it themselves more and find it a useful managerial tool.

HCFA will require modest additional resources to implement and operate a health-based payment system.[3] There also would be some costs to plans, because they would be required to provide encounter-level data. This cost would be small for plans that already collect encounter information with diagnoses (this is true of all plans that pay providers on a fee-for-service basis and many plans in which physicians are salaried). Plans that pass on a percentage of the capitation to large provider groups often do not receive complete encounter data from these providers, some of whom may not have data systems able to collect them. However, given enough lead time and the incentive (or sanction) of lower payments if they do not, providers and plans should be able to produce the requisite data. There are clear benefits to plans and their enrollees from having diagnostic information on healthcare encounters: basic diagnostic information about the burden of illness among their beneficiaries should enable plans and providers to improve care management. HCFA will need an auditing program (similar to the auditing of discharge diagnoses in hospitals) to monitor and sanction systematic over-reporting.[4] We imagine that under-reporting would soon be corrected by plans. To avoid large discontinuities, a phase-in schedule would be sensible, in which initially only part of a plan's payment would be based on its health-based case mix.

The concern that adequate expertise and experience do not exist is much allayed by recent initiatives by Medicaid programs to begin implementing health-based payments. Maryland, Colorado, and other state Medicaid programs are in various phases of implementing diagnostically-based payment systems (see Kronick and Dreyfus 1997 for a description of the Medicaid efforts). And Newhouse et al. (1997) argue that the state-of-the-art has developed sufficiently over the last few years to make trying widespread implementation of diagnostically adjusted payment systems feasible and sensible.

Devote Adequate Resources to Research and Testing to Ensure That Beneficiary Information Meets Needs

The second most important thing to focus on is getting the information provided to beneficiaries to be as comprehensive and clear as possible. Considerable effort is already going into this under the BBA mandate. The contributors to this volume have emphasized how important good, clear, comprehensive information is to helping beneficiaries make well-informed choices. Careful and thorough market testing of the information to be provided—of content, format, and delivery media—is extremely important to ensure that beneficiaries will find the information useful and accessible and that it will aid rather than complicate choices.

It is a daunting task to figure out how to provide useful information about health plan choices to 38 million Medicare beneficiaries, who vary widely in literacy levels. Listing benefits and plan rules and procedures is reasonably straightforward, but providing meaningful quality and performance measures is a formidable challenge. The most innovative private employers who have been working on plan comparison and report card information for employees for a number of years are still experimenting to determine the content and style of information presentation that is most useful. Unfortunately, the public "fishbowl" in which HCFA operates does not lend itself well to experimentation, especially to experiments that fail.

Our suggestions for progress here are not innovative but are worth repeating: HCFA should increase its investment in research on measuring and reporting information that is useful to consumers and should work intensively and collaboratively with beneficiaries and plans to continuously improve information collection and dissemination. The cost of doing this well is small in relation to the cost of producing and distributing information to beneficiaries; the price of not doing it well is high.

Given the present paucity of information and the fact that many beneficiaries do not even know that Medicare HMOs operate in their area, we expect information about zero and low premium plans to have a significant impact on HMO enrollment for people without Medigap and to encourage even high-risk beneficiaries to try HMOs that get good quality and satisfaction ratings, especially if guaranteed annual open enrollment assures the possibility of future access to Medigap coverage. Providing really helpful and comprehensive information could have a significant impact on risk selection. Even if only a minority of beneficiaries were to use the comparative information and take it into consideration in choosing among managed care plans and Medigap insurers, this might provide a powerful incentive to insurers and plans to pay serious attention to their ratings.

Include Medigap in the Information and Coordinated Open Enrollment Under the Same Rules as Medicare+Choice Plans, Including a Common Premium Rating System

The biggest hurdle to including Medigap in the various reforms and improvements to the Medicare system is likely to be resistance from Medigap insurers who fear that their autonomy and profits could be reduced. Medigap insurers will resist losing their right to refuse coverage and being put into more direct competition with HMOs, fearing that they may lose market share to HMOs and have their profit margins squeezed.

At first glance, requiring Medigap to guarantee enrollment at least once per year might seem likely to increase adverse selection against Medigap policies, by increasing access to such policies by the sick. But because most of the sick already have Medigap policies, the actual effect might well be the reverse: namely to give peace of mind to the sick who want to join an HMO that they will be able to regain their Medigap coverage if they discover that they are dissatisfied with managed care.

Require Standardized Marketing Information and Format

Developing a standard format for marketing information would be fairly simple and low cost, and would be very helpful to efforts to compile comparative information charts. Marketing materials are already reviewed, so established procedures exist for checking compliance.

Gather Information on Plan Marketing Impact and Reasons for Not Enrolling in Plans

The only new marketing activity directed at risk selection that HCFA is now considering is to ask plans to make it clear in their marketing materials that disabled Medicare beneficiaries, not just seniors, are eligible to enroll and are welcome. We propose that HCFA play a more proactive role and find out from Medicare beneficiaries whether they believe that plans would welcome them, and whether those who investigate managed care but decide against enrolling have been dissuaded by plans. The costs of running the proposed focus groups and surveys should be modest; abundant expertise is available and this is an efficient and relatively inexpensive way of testing market response. The likely effect on risk selection depends on the unknown extent to which selective marketing is a causal factor and HCFA's ability to devise appropriate corrective actions. Given the potential, the modest costs would seem well worth bearing, at least on an experimental basis.

Offer an Independent Enrollment Broker

Many health plans would resist losing direct control over the enrollment process if independent brokers were to handle enrollment. Some observers of HCFA's unsuccessful attempts to establish competitive bidding demonstrations first in Baltimore and then in Denver have suggested that HMOs were more worried by the enrollment broker feature of the demonstration than by other components more directly linked to competitive bidding. The BBA directs HCFA to conduct a demonstration of the enrollment broker concept. We think that reducing the ability of health plans to directly influence enrollment would have a substantial effect on the extent of risk selection. However, given opposition from plans, the BBA authorization for a demonstration, and some uncertainty about how best to implement a broker function, probably the best that can be expected over the next few years is a well-planned and implemented demonstration project.

Reduce the Diversity of Supplementary Benefit Packages

President Clinton's 1998 budget proposal required partial standardization of the supplementary benefits HMOs offer Medicare beneficiaries. This was not included in the BBA, so implementing this change would require empowering legislation. HMOs would resist restrictions on their freedom to tinker with their benefit packages. On the other hand, standardization of Medigap packages was achieved with relatively little contention, providing a positive precedent. It would be straightforward to accomplish: HCFA would need to survey the range of supplementary benefits offered by HMOs around the country and then, for certain benefits, choose a small number of levels (probably two or three) that may be offered. For example, HMOs might be allowed to offer drug benefits at specified high or low levels. This limitation in diversity would make comparisons easier, but would still potentially leave very large numbers of different plans available in a single market.

Implement Additional Requirements on Plans with Respect to Care for Disabled and Other High-Need Beneficiaries

HCFA is investigating whether disabled beneficiaries are adequately served in HMOs. Twelve large plans have been surveyed to identify "best practices" in catering to the special needs of disabled enrollees. This initiative is still in the analysis and planning stage and is more likely to result in recommendations to plans than requirements.

There would likely be opposition to additional prescriptions and requirements for providing care as involving an inappropriate level of intervention and regulation by HCFA. However, HCFA has a responsibility as a major purchaser of healthcare for Medicare beneficiaries to ensure that their needs will be well served by contracting HMOs. HCFA should work with private sector purchasers, HMOs, and accrediting organizations such as NCQA to arrive at a broad-based consensus on reasonable and appropriate purchasing standards. Going beyond screening criteria when plans apply to participate in Medicare, ongoing monitoring and enforcing compliance with quality of care requirements would be difficult and increasingly costly as the number of plans participating in Medicare increases. And the arguments against reviews of a sample of enrollee deaths to try to establish which were preventable are quite predictable. However, these reviews are routine in hospitals and are potentially beneficial for quality of care.

Survey Disenrollees Who Switch to Fee-for-Service, Monitor the Costs of Their Care, and Consider Penalties to Plans Who "Shed" High-Cost Beneficiaries

The costs of surveying of disenrollees would obviously depend on the frequency and size of the surveys and the method used for carrying them out. If, as suggested in Chapter 8, a short questionnaire could be administered routinely as part of the disenrollment process, costs would be modest. HCFA has all the data needed for monitoring healthcare costs of beneficiaries who disenroll into fee-for-service, so tracking these costs should not be problematic. However, plans would strongly protest any move to make them financially responsible for disenrollees. And if plans believe that high-need beneficiaries have a higher propensity to disenroll for reasons unrelated to the quality of plan service, sanctions would make even the best plans more leery of enrolling them. It might also be difficult to get legislative approval, but the equity and cost implications of disenrollment caused by sick beneficiaries being pushed out by plans are serious enough to warrant considering this proposal.

When the papers upon which several of the chapters in this book were discussed by policymakers and commentators in April 1988, the feasibility of implementing the proposals was on the minds of many. Bruce Vladeck, who was just finishing his term as administrator of HCFA, cautioned that health plans, like most organizations, resist change. Even change that brings improvements is resisted because it requires additional work from people who are already over-stretched and because many people prefer to avoid

unfamiliar situations. So implementing changes involves overcoming inertia and dealing with complaints and resistance. On the other hand, passage
of the BBA has ushered in a period of change and reform in the Medicare
program. Although many activities are competing for attention within HCFA,
the reforms are also creating an environment that is more tolerant of changes.
There is a need to proceed boldly and swiftly, taking full advantage of the
period of fluidity. After 2002, when the BBA is supposed to be fully implemented, plan managers (and others) will doubtless have had enough change
and the window of opportunity will have closed.

CONCLUSION

Increased enrollment of Medicare beneficiaries in HMOs has the potential
to improve quality and access to care for Medicare beneficiaries as well as
reduce the rate of growth of Medicare expenditures. However, this potential
will only be realized if HMOs are rewarded for quality and efficiency, and
not for risk selection.

Fixing the payment system to reward health plans for serving the disabled and chronically ill must be part of the solution. No matter what actions are taken to inhibit "skimming" and encourage high-risk beneficiaries
to try HMOs, if plans lose money when they cater to those in need of care,
they will not orient their systems of care to high-need people. If we want
plans to organize delivery systems to be responsive to the chronically
ill and those most in need, they must be paid commensurately with the
expected healthcare needs of their enrollees. HCFA's current intentions to
begin health-based payment using diagnostic information from inpatient
hospital stays is a useful beginning but should be quickly followed by an
expansion to ambulatory diagnoses as well. Further, HCFA should take the
relatively easy and likely quite effective step of paying health plans for
providing high quality terminal care and should consider proposals for
blended systems of partially capitated and partially fee-for-service reimbursement.

An effective system of health-based payment is necessary, but not sufficient, to create a marketplace in which plans are rewarded for quality and
efficiency. To make a market of competing health plans produce positive
results, beneficiaries need good information about quality and outcomes in
competing plans; a well-ordered and understandable set of choices from
which to choose; reassurance that all plans will produce at least a minimally
acceptable level of quality; accurate marketing materials; responsive and
accessible grievance procedures; and negative consequences for plans from
which high-need members disproportionately disenroll.

Beneficiaries cannot, by themselves, create a market that works. The
theory of managed competition suggests that third parties, or sponsors, are

needed to regulate the interactions of consumers and health plans to ensure that physicians and hospitals and the health plans they join and create are rewarded for serving well those most in need of care. Employers can and in some measure do regulate the interactions of employees and health plans. But only the government can perform these activities on behalf of Medicare beneficiaries.

At the same time that many Republicans in Congress are fond of lambasting HCFA for being bureaucratic and unresponsive, they have imbued HCFA with the responsibility and some of the authority to make a market of competing health plans produce good results for beneficiaries and taxpayers. HCFA faces many challenges in accomplishing this task: the fishbowl in which it operates inhibits innovation and experimentation; the difficulty faced by all large governmental organizations in redeploying internal resources and finding and rewarding good performers; the ready access of aggrieved health plans and providers to Congress and the courts, and the technical difficulties of figuring out how to collect, measure, and communicate information that effectively summarizes the many dimensions of health plan performance. However, to say that the task is difficult is not to say it is impossible. We hope that the material presented in this book will further understanding of the tasks ahead and perhaps facilitate their accomplishment.

NOTES

1. Economists draw a distinction between "avoidance," which obeys the letter of the law, but uses loopholes to get around the intent of the law, and "evasion," which is illegal.
2. Option J covers 50 percent of the cost of prescription drugs after a $250 deductible, up to an annual limit of $3,000.
3. HCFA's main tasks would be to produce county-level estimates of case mix; estimate and adjust for increased intensity of diagnostic reporting that is expected when HMOs are paid based on diagnoses (including auditing HMO reported diagnostic information); process the HMO-generated encounter data; and produce case-mix weights for each plan.
4. A different technical problem is raised by the increased intensity of diagnostic reporting that is expected when plans are paid based on diagnosis. Just as adjustments for "DRG creep" were needed after the introduction of the DRG system, adjustments for "diagnosis creep" or "diagnosis discovery" will be needed and should be expected after HMOs start getting paid based on diagnosis.

REFERENCES

Dallek, G. 1997. "Medicare Managed Care: Securing Beneficiary Protections." Families USA Foundation. www.families.org , March 1998.

Kronick, R., and A. Dreyfus. 1997. *The Challenge of Risk Adjustment for People with Disabilities: Health-Based Payment for Medicaid Programs; a Guide for State Medicaid Programs, Providers and Consumers.* Princeton, NJ: Center for Health Care Strategies.

Newhouse, J., M. B. Buntin, and J. Chapman. 1997. "Risk Adjustment and Medicare: Taking a Closer Look." *Health Affairs* 16 (5): 26–43.

INDEX

About the Authors

Richard Kronick, Ph.D., is an associate professor in the department of family and preventive medicine at the University of California, San Diego. His research focuses on healthcare financing problems. He has developed risk-adjusted payment systems that are being used by state Medicaid programs to pay health plans for persons with disabilities. In 1993–94 he was a senior health policy advisor in the Clinton administration, where he contributed to the design of the administration's healthcare reform proposal. In the late 1980s, he co-authored, with Alain Enthoven, a proposal to achieve universal coverage in the United States and contributed to the development of the theory of "managed competition."

Joy de Beyer, D.Phil., received her doctorate in economics from Oxford University. She has worked as a health economist in the World Bank, providing policy advice and managing funding and technical support to the Ministries of Health in Zimbabwe and Namibia. She worked on this book while holding a post of adjunct assistant professor in the department of family and preventive medicine at the University of California, San Diego.

About the Contributors

Gerard Anderson, Ph.D., is the director of the Center for Hospital Finance and Management, Johns Hopkins Medical Institutions, co-director of the Program for Medical Technology and Practice Assessment, professor and associate chair of health policy and management, Johns Hopkins University School of Hygiene and Public Health, professor of international health and professor of medicine, Johns Hopkins University School of Medicine. He teaches graduate level courses in organization, financing and delivery, comparative health insurance systems, health economics, and health policy.

Tony Dreyfus has been with the Medicaid Working Group at the Boston University School of Public Health since 1993. He has worked primarily on rate setting for Medicaid beneficiaries with disability or chronic illness and has developed with Richard Kronick the Disability Payment System, a classification of diagnoses to set health-based rates for Medicaid beneficiaries. He earned his master's degree in planning from MIT.

Sontine Kalba, BA, is a research analyst at the National Bureau of Economic Research in Stanford, California.

Mark McClellan, M.D., Ph.D., is an assistant professor of economics at Stanford University, an assistant professor of medicine at Stanford Medical School, and an internist in the department of medicine at Stanford University Hospital. His research interests include evaluating the cost and outcome effects of alternative medical treatment choices, the cause and consequences of technologic change in healthcare, and the relationship between health and economic outcomes.

Mark Merlis is a senior fellow at the Institute for Health Policy Solutions, an independent organization in Washington, D.C., that studies healthcare access, cost, quality, and financing issues. Previously he was a senior health policy analyst at the Congressional Research Service, Library of Congress, and an administrator in the Maryland Medicaid program.

Thomas Rice, Ph.D., is professor and chair of the department of health services at the UCLA School of Public Health. He is also editor of the journal *Medical Care Research and Review.* His interests include Medicare reform, physician payment, cost containment, and assessing competitive and regulatory strategies in health policy. Dr. Rice's book *The Economics of Health Reconsidered* was published by Health Administration Press in 1998.